To my parents, who taught me how to make lemonade out of lemons. Without their selfless love, support, confidence, and guidance, I would not have the motivation and determination to achieve my goals. Thank you for your faith in me. I love you.

To my younger sister, Alaina, my best friend, who showed me how to love life; to stop and smell the flowers; to take one day at a time, and to stop looking for too many tomorrows. Thank you for always knowing just what to say. I love you.

To Shannon: Thank you for becoming so involved in diabetes to know how I feel and for trying to step into my shoes. Thank you for your support and understanding and your dedication to helping children. I love you.

To Karey, my partner in crime; to Scott, the craziest person in my life; to Kyle, my friend for 21 years…I love you all!

To Anne, Hope, Kim, Linda, Kathi, Sue, and Beverly…a funny thing about diabetes, you meet the best people along the way! Thank you for all your help.

GROWING U WITH DIA ES

What Children Want Their Parents to Know

ALICIA M^cAULIFFE

CHRONIMED PUBLISHING

Growing Up with Diabetes: What Children Want Their Parents to Know © 1998 by Alicia McAuliffe

Library of Congress Cataloging-in-Publication Data
McAuliffe, Alicia
Growing up with diabetes / by Alicia McAuliffe

       p.   cm.

Includes index.

ISBN 1-56561-150-0; $10.95

Acquiring Editor: Jeff Braun
Editor: Alice Kelly
Cover Design: Maclean & Tuminelly
Text Design & Production: David Enyeart
Art/Production Manager: Claire Lewis
Printed in the United States

Published by
Chronimed Publishing
P.O. Box 59032
Minneapolis, MN 55459-0032

10   9   8   7   6   5   4   3   2   1

Notice: Consult Health Care Professional
Readers are advised to seek the guidance of a licensed physician or health-care professional before making changes in health-care regimens, since each individual case or need may vary. This book is intended for informational purposes only and is not for use as an alternative to appropriate medical care. While every effort has been made to ensure that the information is the most current available, new research findings, being released with increasing frequency, may invalidate some data.

CONTENTS

FOREWORD by Kim Starrett Monroe, M.A., R.D., C.D.E VII

PARENT TO PARENT IX

INTRODUCTION XI

CHAPTER 1 Diabetes "Hurts" Parents More Than Kids 2

CHAPTER 2 Education and Attitude: Equal Partners 20

CHAPTER 3 Getting on with Life 42

CHAPTER 4 The Importance of Social Involvement and Support 54

CHAPTER 5 Working Through Frustrations 68

CHAPTER 6 A Declaration of Independence 84

APPENDIX 1 Diabetes Organizations and Resources 99

APPENDIX 2 Juvenile Diabetes Foundation Chapters 101

INDEX 107

Hindsight is 20/20. How many times have you thought or said that to yourself? Or how about this one: If only I knew then what I know now. Everyone has said this at least once! And I would bet these phrases are used most frequently in our role as parents!

No one offers a professional degree or program of study to become a parent. There are parenting courses, but no career-path study courses. Yet it is our most important role. There is no single course on medicine or nursing or engineering, yet we expect to be good parents with only experience as our guide.

I am a parent of two small children, and I seek out every tidbit on parenting. I entertain the same thoughts that my parents tell me were once theirs: Why don't my children listen? Why don't they understand that I want what is best for them and I know best? Like most people, I am more relaxed or have become more skilled with my second child, because I learned by experience with my first child. Experience is wonderful (though frustrating and painful at times). Resources such as self-help books on parenting are great.

I do not have a child with diabetes (yet), but since I have diabetes there is a chance that one or both of my children could develop it. If that happens, I will seek out a resource like *Growing*

Up with Diabetes. This is especially true because, as someone with diabetes, I am sure I would try to hold my children to the mold of my personal experience. My children are not me. They are male and they have different personalities and ways of handling things.

This book is a fabulous and easy tool to use. We parents are reminded to walk in the shoes of our children, to seek to understand their point of view, to build a trusting relationship, and to aid in guiding our children. Although the author of this book is not a parent, she has plenty to say to parents. Alicia McAuliffe is a very special person. She is young and energetic and relates easily to children and teens. Having worked with Alicia, I have seen how children are at ease with her and seek to walk in her shoes. She is a super role model. While Alicia relates well with children, she is very mature and is equally at ease with parents. She has exquisite communication skills. She listens, actively listens. She seeks to understand before giving advice or counsel.

I am excited that this book is available to parents. Anyone who has met Alicia has reaped the benefits of her skill and experience. Now many, many more will enjoy those same benefits. Her experience helps to guide children, teens, and families to healthier frames of mind living with diabetes. This book is an invaluable, timeless tool with a clear message to seek to understand, seek out help, reach out to others, and help your child reach out.

PARENT TO PARENT

Elizabeth and John McAuliffe

Even though we were aware of this book and somewhat informed of its contents, upon reading it in its entirety, we must say this is the book all parents who have children with diabetes must read.

Alicia was first diagnosed at age 11 by me, her mother. All the symptoms were there—thirst, urination, and blurred vision. At first I was in denial and put the blame on stress or a virus. When the symptoms continued, Alicia was checked and the verdict was in—diabetes. Not my little girl! I had nursed her forever, three years to be exact. She ate all the right homemade food, had sun and fresh air. What could we have done differently? This is the child that had barely ever been bothered by an ear infection. We wracked our brains as to how we could have done this to her. We feared the same for her sister. We feared for her future as well as ours. How could fate be so cruel? After a river of tears and a comfortable grieving period, we knew it was sink or swim.

Alicia seemed okay with her new regimen; we were the restless ones. We took her lead, though, one day at a time. Although still guilt-ridden, we educated ourselves, our family and friends, as well as the entire school about the ins and outs, and literally the ups and downs of diabetes. But of all the books and magazine articles we read, not a single one let us see through her eyes.

And no matter how many times we jabbed ourselves with her needles, we never felt what she felt.

Growing Up with Diabetes took a long time, a lot of maturing and educating, and a lot of soul searching. We are happy to see that it is now written. And by the grace of God and Alicia, we are finally absolved of our guilt and feel only pride.

Remember when your child was diagnosed with diabetes? No doubt you and your family received an overwhelming amount of information about diabetes from nurse educators, dietitians, doctors, and books. You were given all the facts about managing your child's diabetes from a clinical aspect. However, the social and emotional aspect of diabetes, which is equally as important to the health and well-being of your child, was probably under-emphasized. *Growing Up with Diabetes* fills this gap. It gives you an opportunity to understand and relate to your child as he or she grows up with diabetes.

This book is written from my perspective; I am a 21-year-old chiropractic student who has had diabetes for over 10 years. It's about dealing with the social and emotional aspects of diabetes. Importantly, this book is not a medical book. It does not provide advice or details of how to manage the clinical day-to-day aspects of diabetes. If you need medical information about the physiology of diabetes or instructions on insulin dosing, testing equipment, and the like, please consult a physician, certified diabetes educator, or reference book. (A number of excellent resources are suggested in the appendix.)

Why listen to what I have to say about diabetes? First of all, this book is a compilation of insights and advice from the many children, teens, and parents I have counseled. Ever since I was diagnosed with diabetes at the age of 11, I have committed myself to promoting a sense of normalcy and hopefully setting an example for children, young adults, and their families who live with diabetes.

REACHING OUT

My "formal" experience with the psychosocial aspects of adolescence and diabetes began six years ago when I initiated a counseling, classroom, and faculty education program in Albany, New York. Later I became a peer counselor, at Control Diabetes Services, Inc., a diabetes education center, and then at Diabetes Workshop, Inc. For five years I have worked with The Sugar Free Gang, a support group for young children with diabetes. And two years ago I started Kaleidoscope, an activity group for teenagers with diabetes.

I have been a speaker at many professional diabetes-related events. I represented New York State for the American Diabetes Association, lobbying in Washington, D.C., for insurance coverage of diabetes education and medical supplies. I was Northeast Regional Youth Advisor for the American Diabetes Association for two years, and in 1994 was a United States representative at the International Camp for Diabetic Teenagers in Linkoping, Sweden.

All of this led me to start the Circle of Life Camp, Inc., a not-for-profit camp for children and young adults with diabetes. As founder, president, and director of the camp, I host 60 campers each summer for a week in New York's Adirondack mountains, with a volunteer medical staff that includes nurse-certified diabetes educators and physicians. The campers enjoy sports, crafts, and activities while sharing their knowledge, experiences, and concerns about diabetes and adolescence.

SMOOTHING THE WAY

It is my hope that *Growing Up with Diabetes* will make diabetes management less of a battle between you and your child during adolescence. With proper education and communication, your child will be healthier: emotionally, socially, and physically. And, hopefully, you will be able to ease some of your fears about diabetes and the emotional roller coaster you may experience.

Chapter 1 starts off with the emotions parents feel when their children are diagnosed with diabetes. Guilt, anger, and sorrow are normal for parents but need to be absolved in order for you to successfully facilitate the management of your child's diabetes. Children are more accepting and do not have the same ill feelings and fears as adults have about diabetes. You need to focus your energy on managing your child's diabetes instead of your own negative feelings about the condition.

In Chapter 2, you will learn that diabetes education is important for many reasons. Not only does it help in day-to-day management practices, but it helps the family assimilate diabetes into the family, creating a supportive and understanding atmosphere. Education will build a positive attitude for your family, which will transcend to your child's emotional development. Education promotes the acceptance, responsibility, social confidence, and physiological well-being of your child.

Chapter 3 emphasizes the importance of making your child's life as normal as possible. Diabetes should not be the focus of your child's life. Children with diabetes should be interested and involved in all school and extracurricular activities in which children without diabetes participate. A normal environment for your child will foster acceptance of diabetes, which will produce positive emotional and social development.

Chapter 4 explains the unsurpassing value of children with diabetes interacting with each other. Camps, support groups, and fundraising activities are ideal places for children to meet friends with the same concerns, problems, and fears. This social involvement promotes acceptance, support, and confidence for children, which is a therapeutic, irreplaceable experience.

Next, in Chapter 5, you will learn how to manage the inevitable hassles of diabetes. Outside forces are first discussed. For instance, you have probably already experienced the frustration of dealing with misinformed people who unintentionally discriminate against people with diabetes. Uneducated school officials can also be a problem. Then, there are the frustrations of trying to control diabetes; they can be very upsetting. Adolescence is a difficult time to achieve ideal glucose control. Education helps both you and your child cope with the emotional roller coaster of diabetes management.

As you may already know, the power struggle for independence during adolescence can be taxing for parents and kids. Chapter 6 emphasizes that children should assume more responsibility for their diabetes management. It also covers the obstacles that you may encounter as your child matures. With the proper education, social environment, and support, children can become more confident, and emotionally stable, and, as a result, better able to accept care for their own diabetes.

Finally, the appendices list a variety of resources for both you and your child, including helpful books and publications on diabetes management as well as the local chapters of the Juvenile Diabetes Foundation International (JDF).

POWERFUL WORDS

Throughout this book, I refer to diabetes as a chronic condition, rather than a disease. Diabetes is technically a disease. However, the word disease implies sickness. People with diabetes are not sick. If they manage their diabetes properly, they are just as healthy, or possibly healthier, than people without diabetes. That's because people with diabetes usually are more conscious of their food, exercise regularly, and have regular medical exams.

When I talk to children about diabetes, I am especially careful when choosing my words. I use the words chronic condition instead of disease. The word disease is especially intimidating to children, connoting something terminal. When I was diagnosed, and told I had a disease, I was frightened. The word disease meant that I would die soon, that I had a time limit! And when rumors spread around school that I had a disease, my classmates were afraid and treated me differently. They didn't talk to me because they were afraid they would catch my disease. Other kids were extra nice because they felt sorry for me.

Yes, there are many complications associated with diabetes. The risk of eye, kidney, and nerve damage is higher in people with diabetes; however, if diabetes is well controlled, complications can be avoided, delayed, or minimized. Beginning good management habits during childhood will lead the way to a healthier, happier life for your child.

GROWING UP WITH DIABETES

What Children Want Their Parents to Know

Chapter 1

Diabetes "Hurts" Parents More Than Kids

"As individual as the disease is for the child, the experience is individual for the parents."

"I know when people ask me if I'm OK or if I'm allowed to eat something, they're being nice, but it gets on your nerves after a while."

KAYLA, 15

> "What seems nasty, painful, evil can become a source of beauty, joy and strength, if faced with an open mind. Every moment is a golden one for him who has the vision to recognize it as such."
>
> HENRY MILLER

Listen to your little ones, and you will learn volumes. Their quiet little voices will ring loudest in your ears. Their tiny hands will show you strength, and their minds, the wisdom of Solomon. They are loving and trusting and lay blame on no one. I am giving you a look at the other side of diabetes—growing up with it. Allowing you, a parent, to walk in the shoes of your child. I know from my parents how challenging it is to raise a child, let alone a child with diabetes. It is devastating to be faced with the realization that diabetes will now be a part of your family's life. It helps to know that you and your family are not alone.

My name is Alicia McAuliffe and I am 21 years old. I was diagnosed with diabetes at the age of 11. Sound familiar? Since then, I have committed myself to promoting a sense of normalcy and hopefully set an example for young adults and parents struggling to cope with adolescence and diabetes. I am the founder, camp director, and president of the Circle of Life Camp Inc., a not-for-profit camp for children and young adults with diabetes, and have counseled and facilitated numerous support activities for children with diabetes and their families.

All parents who have children with diabetes have their own stories of how diabetes became part of their lives, and how and when their child was diagnosed. That moment is frozen and imprinted into your brain; you own it and re-live it daily, consciously or unconsciously. Your child might have been hospitalized because she was in ketoacidosis, or your child was in trouble at school because she wasn't doing well or kept using the bathroom. Or it may have been a fluke; your child may have had the flu and was diagnosed during a routine visit to the doctor's office. Or as Heather, age 15, says, "It runs in my family." At my camp we had an informal discussion about how campers were diagnosed with diabetes. Ironically, over half a dozen campers were diagnosed on their birthday!

All families have their own unique story, but every parent has similar feelings about diabetes. I have yet to meet a parent who says, "I think diabetes is great. I'm so happy that my daughter was diagnosed." One wise parent said, "There is a reason for everything, and God must have thought that my daughter was a strong enough person to handle this, to let her get diabetes."

"I felt that our life was a nightmare when my son was diagnosed," said one of my camper's parents, which sums up most parent's feelings. In working with children and their families, I have found that the parents have more difficulty accepting and adjusting to diabetes than the child. You blame yourself or deny the matter entirely. Some become overprotective and smother the child. You keep asking yourself, "What did I do wrong?" "What could I have done to prevent it?" As one parent said, "At first you feel like your entire life has been taken away and you are a slave to diabetes." You are angry at the world and become more focused on your child's diabetes than your child as a person. This is a normal stage. Why wouldn't you react this way? You want your children to be perfect, free from sorrow or pain. You would do anything to shield them from harm. Diabetes shatters all of this. You would trade places with your child in a blink of an eye. But no matter how much you pray and wish, diabetes won't go away. The next best thing is to deal with diabetes in a healthy way, so your child has a normal life and diabetes becomes less of an enemy that you are both fighting.

You will always remember special events in your child's life. Her birth and the day she was diagnosed with diabetes will be the forerunners. I remember the day I was diagnosed, or, should I say, when my beta cells were declared officially dead. That's what I thought it was: a funeral. That morning we had just buried my father's mother. My father did not cry then. However, when the doctor told my parents that the nurse was taking me into the next room and that he would stay and talk to them about my diabetes, my father started to cry. At that time I couldn't understand why my father, who didn't cry when he saw his mother buried a few hours before, was crying over a few of my dead beta cells. My mother held me on her lap, shaking, as if she thought the doctor was going to snatch me away. He didn't, but fate did. I was thinking to myself, I'm not dying. It's not like they told my parents I had only days to live. Things could be a lot worse. So what's the big deal? I'll take a few shots. The word "shots" rang in my parents' ears like bullets fired from the doctor's mouth.

ADJUSTING TO DIABETES

The next few weeks were a small adjustment for me. The next few years were a *huge* adjustment for my parents. But that's natural. Children are able to adjust to things more quickly than adults. Children live on a day-to-day basis. Children's courage is always a mystery to adults; where they find it no one knows. Parents, however, are always projecting into the future, worrying about what may or may not be, so their fear is heightened. My mother told me that some of her first questions to the doctor were, "Can she have kids?" and "Will she be able to go to college?" instead of asking questions about the next day or the following week, when I would return to school. My first thought was "Will I be able to go to Amy's birthday party on Friday?" My parents were worried about the long-term impact of diabetes and how it would change my life and my family's life. I was worried that I wouldn't be back for my school field trip next week. I'm not saying that every child will have the same reaction to diabetes. However, it is safe to say that children are more accepting than parents.

When some children are diagnosed, they are angry at the world and feel sorry for themselves, or deny the fact that they have diabetes, just as parents do. And they should be allowed to feel this way. Having diabetes is not a party. But staying angry, feeling sorry for yourself, or denying diabetes does not help matters. Children want to be normal, and diabetes makes them "different." Parents need to be sensitive to their child's feelings and to listen to her. Although diabetes is overwhelming for you, the parents, and you may not be ready to help your child, it is imperative that you do. It is imperative that you listen to your child's concerns, questions, and feelings at the time of diagnosis and also during adolescence and her adult life. Children lean on their parents for support and encouragement, and for a child living with diabetes, this is even more important. You taught your child how to crawl, walk, and talk; now you must teach her to live, to survive, and to thrive.

As a parent, you need to confront your own emotions of guilt, anger, and sorrow before you can successfully facilitate the management of your child's condition. You need to realize that there is nothing that you as a parent could have done to prevent diabetes. And stop thinking, "if only I could have!" You need to focus your energy on how you can help your child now. You need to accept your child's diabetes in order to help her.

Parents live and breathe diabetes, but you need to remember yourself also, or you may have other family conflicts. You need to take time out for yourself and your spouse. You should continue your job, hobbies, and activities with friends. If you feel overwhelmed by the emotional stress of diabetes, seek professional help and/or talk to other parents with similar feelings. You need to deal with your feelings and emotions, because your child will need to lean on you for support.

Children are told by their parents what is right and wrong, when to go to bed, what and when to eat, and how to live their lives. So to have a parent give three cookies for a snack, "and no more because dinner will be in a few hours," is not a major lifestyle change to a child. As an adult, you have your own routine and habits with no parent to whom you must answer. It is more difficult to fit diabetes into an adult lifestyle and to relearn a new routine while unlearning old habits. I was giving myself injections and had the "check the sugar" routine and my meal plan down within a month, never missing a dance or piano lesson. But it took my mother six months to be able to watch me do an injection, the injection that was to be my life support in addition to the normal life-sustaining requirements of air, water, and food. These are the things that haunt parents daily.

The helplessness of all parents is at times overwhelming as well as depressing. Strange things go through your mind, I was told. My parents worried about being stranded somewhere on some deserted island (which was pretty unlikely), without food or insulin, and they calculated how long they could hold on to me. Helplessness and losing control are scary to the ones that are to be a child's strength and protectors.

Don't get me wrong; my parents were great. They were very supportive and understanding and tried never to let me see how upset they were. Actually, it was only a few years ago that I mentioned noticing them going out less frequently when I was younger, and told them that I knew how upset they really were. That's why I did what I was supposed to do to control my diabetes when I was younger: so that they would stop worrying. But parents never stop worrying. Even now, after 10 years, when my mother is talking about my diabetes or sees that I'm not feeling well because I'm low, tears fill her eyes. Never underestimate the hurt a parent feels, it is deep and lasting.

When a child mistakenly gives herself a painful morning in-

jection into a muscle and it starts to bleed, she is outside playing with friends 10 minutes later and has forgotten about the injection and the pain. But you are still thinking about the morning
injection as you are tucking her into bed at night. It's important
to remember that diabetes "hurts" parents more than the child.

About six months ago, I became very ill with a head cold,
high fever, and stomach virus. (In the 10 years I have had diabetes, I had never seen the inside of a hospital, not even when I
was diagnosed.) When I was sick, I became so weak from dehy-
dration (I was spilling ketones, although my sugar was only 200
mg/dl [11.1 mmol/L*]), my parents brought me to the hospital. I was admitted into the hospital for two days. The doctors
thought I had meningitis. They took what seemed like 100 blood
samples, X-rays, CAT scans, and a spinal tap. When I had my
spinal tap at 2 a.m., I was exhausted and very weak. When the
doctor started numbing my back before inserting the needle to
draw my spinal fluid, I started to cry and my mother joined me.
By the time the doctor was finished, I had calmed down but my
mother hadn't. She was still crying hysterically. The doctor
leaned over and said to me, "I think that hurt your mother more
than you."

It's important to realize that children notice the sorrow, anger,
and worry that their parents feel. Society in general underesti-
mates a child's intelligence. Most children under the age of nine
with diabetes know about ketoacidosis, what the normal blood-
glucose range is, how to check their blood sugar, and that they

---

*Outside the United States, blood glucose is often measured in millimols per liter
(mmol/L). To convert a test result in mg/dl to mmol/L, simply divide the number
by 18.

need to eat when they are low. This information and vocabulary is quite impressive for such a young age. If children are able to learn this complex information about the medical aspect of diabetes, it is not difficult for them to learn what emotions are associated with their condition. Kyle, age 8, says, "Sometimes my parents are very sad."

ALL IN THE FAMILY

No one lives in isolation, so diabetes affects the entire family. When a family has a child with diabetes, it is common to unintentionally give more attention to the child with diabetes than to children without diabetes. Parents are concerned about the unending list of things the child with diabetes has to remember: what she should be eating, when she needs to check her sugar or take insulin, or if she remembered glucose tablets.

One time my younger sister, Alaina, said to me, "You're lucky. I want diabetes. You get all the attention." I never realized she felt this way, nor did my parents. I felt as if my parents were bothering me when they reminded me of my snack or made a fuss when I was low. You need to set aside time for your children without diabetes and do something special, especially if they are young. My parents started doing this and Alaina stopped wanting diabetes. At 17 years old, my sister reflects, "I felt left out when I was younger. I thought my sister was the lucky one. However, now that I am older and actually understand diabetes, I want to help improve my sister's life and the lives of other people who live with diabetes."

Children with diabetes appreciate and benefit from the support and involvement of their siblings. Rebecca, 11 years old, said, "My sister hides candy." Sarah, age 11, shared, "My brother helps out when I'm low by getting a juice pack." Nicholas, age 12, says "I help my younger sister who also has diabetes with her injections."

My friend, Karey, who has diabetes told me that when she was younger, her mother took her brother out to the store once a month and allowed him to eat as much candy as he wanted. Her mother felt guilty for not keeping sweets in the house and depriving him. (Now that the medical community has realized that candy can be fit into the diabetes regimen, parents can allow their child with diabetes to eat sweets.) I'm not recommending to have your other children binge on candy, but set aside time for them to show them that they are special too.

The key word is "special," not different. All children need to feel special. When I was first diagnosed my wise endocrinologist shared a little untold "secret." He said that, due to the increase in my blood sugar, my brain would benefit and I would become smarter. He told me I would retain information better, my grades would improve, and I would become a much smarter person. Well, it worked! Fact or not, my doctor is a very smart man, and I still feel that this "scientific fact" did me a world of good.

One night at Circle of Life Camp, the campers started putting craft ribbons in one another's hair. Within an hour everyone at camp—boys, and girls, campers, nurses, and counselors—all had ribbons in their hair. We all looked ridiculous and were laughing at one another's hair. But no one felt uncomfortable, self-conscious, or "different." Everyone looked equally ridiculous and felt like they belonged.

Diabetes is a family effort. Other siblings should be educated about diabetes. When my sister Alaina was old enough to understand diabetes, we educated her. She is now actively involved in the Juvenile Diabetes Foundation and the American Diabetes Association. She helps out with support groups for children with diabetes, and she is also a counselor at my camp. Alaina has supported me and helped many other youths overcome negative attitudes about diabetes. She has made them feel special.

It is important that everyone in the house is educated about diabetes, in the event something happens. When I was 15 and my sister 12, she saved my life. During the summer months, my parents would occasionally allow me to sleep later without waking me up to take an injection and eat. My parents left for work in the morning and told my sister to wake me up at 10 o'clock. When my sister tried to wake me, I hit her and began to have a seizure. My sister called my mother and immediately started to rub honey on my gums. About two hours later I finally gained consciousness. I discovered seven people looking over me! Including your other children in diabetes management will make them feel less left out, it will allow them to react in emergency situations, and it fosters a supportive environment for your child with diabetes.

DEALING WITH GUILT

You, as a parent, are entitled to feel angry with the world. You are allowed to feel that diabetes isn't fair: Why did this happen to *my* family, *my* child? You are entitled to feel sorry for yourself and for your child. But many parents also feel guilty. One parent said to me, "I felt hurt and guilty. I felt sorry for my 2 1/2 year old baby. It didn't seem fair!" As a child I understood anger and sorrow, but I never understood why my parents felt guilty. It is not as if my parents gave me food laced with beta cell destroying toxins, or said, "Naughty, naughty, I wish diabetes on you," or had direct control over me developing diabetes in *any* way. The only way they could have avoided my diabetes was not to have had me altogether. However, now that I am older, I understand why my parents felt responsible. My parents, as well as many other parents, hold themselves responsible because they love me and are very protective of me. They felt guilty because I couldn't eat what or when or how much I wanted. They felt guilty because I got low and they had no control over it. They felt guilty because I was the one taking injections and pricking my finger, and not them.

The children I have counseled and those who attend my camp would agree with me in saying, as a child with diabetes, I never blamed my diabetes on my parents. It's in my DNA—out of *anyone's* control. I confess that sometimes I did get angry with my mother when she told me I couldn't have a second piece of cake. But all children become upset with their parents when they are not allowed to do what they want, even though it is in the child's best interest. When my parents became more comfortable with my diabetes, they accepted a few higher readings for an extra piece of pizza or cake at a party. And I accepted this as a treat. Other children didn't have to worry about things like this.

You are used to making things "all better" for your children. You lose this control and security when your child has diabetes. This is very frustrating and frightening. You have no choice but to allow nature to take control. When talking to a parent full of anguish, the most common cry of desperation I hear is, "I wish I could take it away from my child!" When a parent says this in tears, I am dumbfounded. I don't think there is an appropriate response to this. It is a normal feeling and reaction of protection. As a person who has grown up with diabetes through adolescence, I can tell you that everything will be okay. I survived, I am a well-adjusted individual who is a productive member of society. I can tell them that I had ups and downs, but with the support of my family, I think I'm a stronger person because of my diabetes. But no matter how much I console a parent, it doesn't ease her desperation. No matter how many times I tell my mother and father that I'm okay, it doesn't help. Parents worry.

You worry even more when your child becomes upset. I know I get frustrated with my diabetes because my numbers are high for no apparent reason, and my parents feel guilty. When I get upset, it is not at them. However, they somehow feel responsible. They feel that it is some inadequacy in their parenting, which it's not. Parents need to realize that children do notice their effort, concern, and support, and appreciate it (although we don't often verbalize that).

A supportive family is the "safety net" for difficult situations. My parents supported, encouraged, and cried with me when I was upset, which was the best therapy. I know my parents were not sure if they were appropriately coping with my diabetes, but I know they were trying their best, which was the perfect way. They were attentive to my feelings and concerns as well as their own, not compromising either one. Children do not come with an instruction book, nor does diabetes. Raising a child with diabetes is a trial-and-error process. Although parents wish there

14

was a "set way" to manage their child's diabetes, there isn't. Families need to find their own way to manage the diabetes regimen—a way that is comfortable for the parents and the child. This is vital to successful diabetes management.

When I was first diagnosed, my mother was convinced that my diabetes would go away and desperately tried to convince the doctor that she was going to find the way how. My doctor looked at her and said, "If Alicia's diabetes goes away, I'll convert to your religion." (We're Catholic, he's Jewish). This was a very final-sounding statement to my mother, and she became angry at the world. Diabetes is final: you just can't have a "touch" of diabetes, and one person cannot have diabetes worse than another person. But, diabetes is not the end of the world either, although it seems so at that time.

Actually, even at the age of 21, I'm not sure my parents have completely accepted the fact that I will have diabetes forever. They are still praying for a miracle. But it is part of me now. Diabetes has made me a stronger, more responsible, mature person. I'm sure my parents still feel sorrow. But I don't. A common reaction people have when they find out that I have diabetes is, "Oh, I'm sorry." My response is, "I'm not." I don't want people to feel sorry for me. All people have problems in their life whether it's health, family, or financial. I could have been diagnosed with a terminal disease, but I was lucky enough to have something that is treatable with medication. There are new treatments available every year, making my life and the lives of others with diabetes a little bit easier. There is nothing that I could say or anyone else could say to absolve these feeling of a parent. But after a while these feelings actually make matters worse, interfering with management of your child's diabetes. Many parents have explained to me that time makes diabetes easier. Now that your child has diabetes, there is nothing you can do to reverse it. You need to focus now on how to best manage your child's diabetes together with your child. You must focus on the present, not dwell on what could or should have been.

SET AN EXAMPLE

Children learn their values and beliefs from their parents. If you feel anger about your child's diabetes or are in denial, your child will likely develop these same feelings. Children learn their attitudes about diabetes. Young children are naive and have an innocence that disappears when fear and anger are instilled. This is not a steadfast rule, and some children do have a negative attitude toward diabetes without parental influence. However, most parents who have a negative attitude toward diabetes will teach it to their children. To help and guide your child, you need to absolve feelings of guilt and anger and any wrongdoing, and focus your energy on the management of your child's diabetes, making your child's life as "normal" as possible. A parent needs to have a more optimistic attitude about diabetes, and see that the condition does not limit their child in any way, including eating. Your child is able to do anything, as long as she fits her diabetes regimen into her schedule. And, most importantly, your child can still aspire to her dreams. This positive thinking will improve the life of your child with diabetes and your family. Your positive parental guidance will decrease the negative attitude of your child and hopefully increase compliance with her diabetes treatment regimen.

Instead of wishing away the diabetes, hating the entire world, or feeling guilty, you must refocus your energy in another direction. Your goal is now to effectively manage your child's diabetes together with your child in a manner that is comfortable for both of you. This collaborative effort will allow optimal social and psychological development of your child. Brace yourself, because you will encounter many obstacles when raising a child with diabetes. Sound overwhelming? The outcome is worth the effort tenfold!

Chapter Summary

"I wish I may, I wish I might!" All the wishing in the world won't make diabetes go away, but facing it together will make it a lot easier. Don't ever give up hope or faith in yourself or your ability to rise above this intruder. Faith and fortitude are what got medical science where it is today—better insulin, better delivery systems, and better control. Treatment for diabetes is not perfect, and there is no cure yet; but together we need to walk those walks, run those miles, and bike our way to a cure. While we are doing all these things, we need to remember to look around and see that we are not alone—there is strength in numbers. We cannot give up the fight with diabetes: our strategies, determination, and continuous education. The feeling of helplessness you and your child feel can and will be overwhelming at times, but join forces together and you will come out victorious.

SOUNDING OFF

What Real Kids Say...

"One of the most aggravating things is to observe someone using their diabetes as a crutch or an excuse, because it gives the impression that people with diabetes have a major handicap."

KAREY, 21

Chapter 2

Education and Attitude: Equal Partners

"When your child becomes older and independent, it is harder for you, as a parent, to keep up with all the new diabetes technology."

"My parents always talk to me about my sugar. I really appreciate when they involve me in diabetes-management decisions."

KRISTEN, 11

"The longer I live, the more I realize
the impact of attitude on life…
I am convinced that life is 10 percent
what happens to me and 90 percent
how I react to it."

CHARLES SWINDOLL

When I was first diagnosed with diabetes, the only information my family had about diabetes was from television and movies. For entertainment purposes, diabetes complications and problems that may arise are greatly exaggerated. For example, in a movie, if a person is dying in the hospital and is given an insulin injection, he instantly becomes super-human and can fight an army of men single-handedly. Or a movie character is diagnosed with diabetes and the following day becomes blind. I now sit back and laugh about the way diabetes is portrayed on television and in the movies. However, before my family and friends were educated about the condition, they expected me to be very sickly based on the information they had learned watching movies. My parents were afraid of me not being able to have children. There are common

misconceptions about diabetes because there is no accurate information circulating throughout the general public. Recently, I
read a newspaper article which stated that people taking a certain
medication may "contract" diabetes. Diabetes is not contagious,
unless the reporters have information that I have not received!

EDUCATE YOUR FAMILY

Diabetes education is very important for your family, your child
with diabetes, your child's school, and the people with whom
your child has frequent contact. Education is a continuous
process. As one parent expressed, "There is never enough education. It is a continuous learning process—you always need to
be kept informed." Education dispels misconceptions about diabetes and may defuse uncomfortable situations that your child
may encounter. Most individuals with diabetes find that well-
meaning family and friends may have a distorted concept of diabetes. The most common misconceptions of diabetes are:
People with the condition are not allowed sugar, including cookies and candy; we can't eat salt; we will go blind, suffer kidney
failure, and lose our appendages. These ideas of diabetes are
what movies glorify and what organizations use when soliciting
money for diabetes research, so the general public is informed on
the extremes of diabetes, rather than day-to-day realities of living with it. I believe diabetes research is vital and understand
organizations' need to use the horrifying side of diabetes to so-
licit money. People do have these tragic complications. But there
are also a great number of people with diabetes who, with the
proper education and support, are very healthy and do not have
these complications.

About three years ago, I took my support-activity group, "Kaleidoscope" (for teenagers with diabetes), ice-skating. An older woman at the counter asked if I was baby-sitting, because I had 10 kids about 12 years old with me. I explained to her that it was a support group for teenagers with diabetes. She made a huge scene by saying, "Oh my gosh, you poor little children. Here, have a free diet soda." We accepted the soda. As she was distributing the soda, I tried to explain to her that we are very healthy and just need to follow a medication regimen, eat health-ily, and exercise. She was shocked when I told her that I also had diabetes. She said, "You look so good for having diabetes for such a long time." She went on to tell me her husband "contracted" diabetes at the age of 50 and died two years later of a heart at-tack. I spent the next hour explaining to the kids how people are misinformed about diabetes and how to handle situations like this that arise, because they were very surprised at the woman's reaction (although they thought it was neat to get a free soda).

This reaction among the general public to diabetes, especially toward children with diabetes, is very common. Moira, 12 years old, says, "I hate when people feel sorry for me and make a big deal." Kristen, age 12, also agrees, "People just don't under-stand."

Despite their despair and fear, my parents educated me about diabetes. Educating me is probably the best thing that my par-ents could have ever done for me (besides finding a cure). After I was diagnosed, I saw a diabetes educator and dietitian with my parents. We subscribed to a few diabetes magazines to keep up to date about new diabetes research, and became involved in the Juvenile Diabetes Foundation and the American Diabetes Association. Whatever my parents learned, I did too. This allowed me to become more independent. I truly believe that education is the key to acceptance, independence, confidence, and compliance to a diabetes regimen. This in turn supports healthy psychological and social development.

EDUCATE YOUR CHILD

When I was diagnosed, I was 11 and mature enough to attend educational sessions with my parents and to understand what my diabetes educators taught. However, the level of information and the language used to educate your child depends on his age and maturity. For example, a few years ago I counseled a very mature, smart 7-year-old girl who was worried that she may have retinopathy in 10 years. She talked with me about ketoacidosis, how much insulin she takes, her sliding scale, and her fear of retinopathy. Adults fear retinopathy; however, I thought it was very unusual for a child to worry about the diabetes eye complication. She was very educated about diabetes and could understand the information and terminology very well. On the other hand, I've also met many children her age whose only involvement in their diabetes management is to prick their finger and wipe their injection site with alcohol. An important thing to remember is that diabetes education should be age-appropriate for your child. As he gets older, provide him with more complex information.

I have found that many families are uneducated about diabetes or have not kept up to date with new diabetes information. Education and updated information are essential for a healthy life with diabetes. I have talked with numerous families that have had trouble with their children rebelling against diabetes. This is very common, but it is even more common in families that have not had proper diabetes education.

Once when I was talking with a mother who was desperate to help her daughter, it became clear to me that the family was in the dark about diabetes. The teenager was doing the bare necessities of management. She was not following a diet plan or carbohydrate counting; she was not adjusting her insulin to accommodate high readings or checking her sugar regularly. This was mostly because her doctor was not informed or did not inform them. The teenager and her family were never told about the 1993 Diabetes Complications and Control Trials. This study concluded that people with diabetes who maintained near-normal glucose levels can avoid or at least delay complications. This is an incentive for people with diabetes to take proper care and to maintain good control. Tight control is different in children, because doctors are concerned with hypoglycemia. And this tight control is not as important in children with diabetes until after puberty. High glucose levels do not have a long-term impact until after puberty. However, if a child is chronically high, he may do poorly in school and not feel well. These chronic high readings may also have an impact on physical development. This information is important to be aware of because it motivates people to comply with their diabetes regimen. If I were not made aware of this information about delaying and possibly avoiding complications, I would be more likely to do only the bare necessities of management. Why would I care about adjusting my insulin according to my sugar readings? Why would I check my sugar at least four times a day, if I were not adjusting my insulin?

Why would I care what my HbA1c was? There would be no purpose in taking multiple daily injections or wearing the insulin pump, if I achieved the same end result with only one injection per day.

If I didn't know that I could eat everything and anything I wanted by fitting the food into my diabetes regimen, I would sneak things such as candy. I have a sweet tooth and love candy. Candy is not healthy for anyone, but I enjoy it and my sugar is normal because I adjust my insulin. I eat frozen yogurt every day (candy and frozen yogurt are my vices). This shocks parents. New information has shown that the carbohydrate content in foods is what affects blood glucose, whether it is fruit, candy, ice cream, or crackers. People are not informed of this information and children are deprived of sweet foods, which is unfair! Of course, sweets are not especially nutritious and should be taken in moderation. Ten years ago when I was diagnosed, I was only allowed to have ice cream once a week, and only if my sugar was "good" during that week. I was unintentionally punished if my sugar was high, because the medical community did not know that it was the amount of carbohydrate in foods that affects glucose levels, rather than the source of the carbohydrate. So, I guess I'm making up for lost time now!

Another important point in education is the way you refer to glucose readings. As a parent you should avoid making value judgments about your child's readings. A reading of 100 mg/dl (5.6 mmol/L) is not a "good" reading, and a reading of 350 mg/dl (19.4 mmol/L) is not "bad." A reading of 100 mg/dl is "normal," while a reading of 350 mg/dl is "high" and reading of 45 mg/dl (2.5 mmol/L) is "low." When labeling a reading as "bad," you inadvertently judge and correlate the reading to the person, and your child feels bad. High readings are sometimes uncontrollable under stressful situations, sickness, and puberty. Your child may be very sensitive about his glucose readings, thinking that they reflect on himself as a person. A glucose reading does not reflect on the type of person an individual is; therefore, it should not be identified with positive or negative meanings. The words, "high," "low," and "normal," however, are neutral words and have a more positive effect on a child's self-image.

Education is just as important for children as it is for their parents. A child who is educated will become more comfortable with himself and his diabetes, and will have more self-confidence. An educated child will understand why he needs to follow his diabetes regimen and be more compliant. An educated child may have fewer psychosocial problems during adolescence because he has an understanding of the condition.

EDUCATE YOUR CHILD'S SCHOOLMATES

Adolescence is a period where social acceptance is important. Amy, 9 years old, said, "All my classmates picked on me and poked fun of my diabetes when I was first diagnosed." When I was first diagnosed, I didn't want anyone to know there was something "wrong" with me. I didn't want to be different or to be treated differently. After I was educated, my parents convinced me that the school nurse and teachers needed to know about my condition, in the event that something happened or because I needed to eat in class. I realized that my friends would eventually find out: If I got low when I was with them and I *had* to get something to eat immediately, my friends would think that something was different. Or if I were to eat in class without a reaction from the teacher, that would also be strange. So I reluctantly told my friends about it.

After the school nurse persuaded me, I did my first classroom presentation with my Pink Panther Book (see Appendix 1) to explain diabetes. The nurse told me that educating my classmates about diabetes would make me feel more comfortable, because I would avoid getting teased. She told me that I should educate them to avoid prejudice against me, so my classmates wouldn't think they could catch diabetes from me or think that I was weird eating a snack at 10 o'clock when no one else was eating. I hesitantly agreed to talk to the class and to my surprise, everyone was interested in diabetes and thought what I did was "neat." Everyone knew about my diabetes and I wasn't embarrassed. I didn't do anything wrong to "get" it. In fact, after I showed everyone my meter and syringe, they wanted to know more. This helped me feel more comfortable with my diabetes and myself. By educating my friends and classmates, I wasn't estranged from anyone and I was still Alicia. Danny, 10 years old, said, "After I told my friends about diabetes, they never paid attention to it."

Informing and educating the people at your child's school is very important. Your diabetes educator can help educate the school, so that your child can assimilate into school more comfortably and with more confidence. Amiee, 11 years old, explained to me, "Before my class was taught about diabetes, everyone thought it was contagious." The basics of diabetes should be explained to the school faculty. The school nurse can also play an important role in educating the faculty if you or your diabetes educator is not able. One parent suggested, "There should be more diabetes education in the schools where there are kids with diabetes attending. Also, written material such as a pamphlet should be distributed to the teacher, explaining the importance of snacks at specific times and hypoglycemia, etc." The importance of scheduled eating times should be stressed to school officials. If your school has two lunch periods, try to request the one that most closely corresponds to your child's regimen. Request a school lunch menu, so that you can choose meals that fit your child's meal plan (and send additional food if required). This will let your child buy lunch at school along with his friends.

Try to assimilate your child's diabetes into the normal school routine. Ask your child's teacher to move snack time closer to your child's snack schedule. Also, ask if you can give the teacher extra food, in case your child forgets his snack or gets low. If your child's class does not have a snack time, then have your child eat his snack quietly at his desk. Do not allow the teacher to single out your child by announcing that, "Mike needs to eat his snack because he has a disease," or send him out of the room to the nurse to eat his snack. Ashley, 12 years old, told me, "My teacher told the class that I had diabetes and no one would talk to me. They stayed away from me." Although the teacher may be well meaning, this unneeded emphasis on your child's diabetes reminds him that he is different. When educating the people at school, explain diabetes clearly, so they are not frightened by it and so they don't exclude your child from field trips and other special events at school.

Explaining what hypoglycemia is and how it should be treated is vital to your child's safety. Chris, 12 years old, told me, "Once, when I got low, the teacher would not let me go to the nurse." Another adolescent, Cori, who is 15 years old, said, "When I got low in class, the teacher said that I do a bad job controlling my diabetes." When your child is low, he should be allowed to go to the nurse, preferably escorted by a friend to ensure that he gets to the nurse's office safely. And the teacher should allow your child to keep extra food in the classroom in the event that he does become low. When your child has a reaction in class, the teacher should not make a huge scene alarming the students. Jeremy, age 10, said, "When I am low in class everyone stays away from me." Educating the school decreases the incidence of prejudicial circumstances your child may encounter with misinformed teachers and school officials, and improves social acceptance. Kimberly, 9 years old, said, "When I got low in class, my friend stuck up for me and told the teacher that I had to go to the nurse's office."

When I was in fifth grade, my classmates and my teachers were aware that I had diabetes and ate snacks at my desk. One day we had a substitute teacher and I assumed that my teacher had informed her that I had diabetes. At 10:30 a.m., I started eating my snack. The substitute teacher saw me eating and scolded me in front of the class and took my snack away. I tried to explain that I was allowed to eat in class because I had diabetes, but she thought I was talking back to her and sent me to the principal's office. I was angry and embarrassed and the school didn't seem to care much. The teacher didn't even apologize. Your child can avoid this by personally telling a substitute teacher at the start of class that you have diabetes and may need to eat in class!

Allow your child to help educate his teacher and classmates and take part in his diabetes care. This will give your child a sense of responsibility over his condition. When I was first diagnosed, my parents and I went into school and explained to my teacher and school officials that I had diabetes and what it entailed. Giving your child some responsibility over their diabetes at a young age—such as pricking their finger, preparing their injection site with alcohol, and assisting in educating his school— paves the way for your child to grow up to be a responsible, independent young adult. During the course of the school year, talk to your child and listen to his feedback on how his diabetes is treated in school. Allow him to make suggestions or reasonable modifications that would make him feel more comfortable with his diabetes at school. Feeling comfortable with his diabetes at school and not being embarrassed about it is one of the largest steps toward acceptance of his condition and compliance to his regimen. As your child matures he will take on more responsibility for controlling his diabetes and educating people about it.

DATING, ADOLESCENCE, AND DIABETES

As your child gets older, an important issue that he will encounter is dating pressures. When a person with diabetes (or a person with any chronic condition) meets someone he is romantically interested in, he doesn't want to scare his potential girlfriend away by telling her that there is something "wrong" with him. I felt this way and was just "friends" with boys. In high school, I was best friends with a boy named Shannon. He knew I had diabetes. He checked his sugar occasionally on my meter, helped me when I was low, and was very educated and supportive of me and my diabetes. One day he asked me out romanti-cally. This shocked me. Beside the fact that he was my best friend, why would he like someone who had something "wrong" with her? He got angry with me and actually opened my eyes. He told me to stop thinking that diabetes was my life, that there was a lot more to me as a person than just that. I had been involved in numerous extra-curricular activities, I was a good student, and I never allowed diabetes to stop me from doing anything. But I always assumed that diabetes was intimidating to people, espe-cially boyfriends or girlfriends. I was very wrong.

Shannon has been a tremendous source of support to me. He keeps glucose tablets in his glove compartment. He carries my diabetes supplies for me when we go skiing. He was at my side in the hospital calming me down. He knows when I'm low before I do and has ridden his bike more than 200 miles to raise money for diabetes. Shannon's support of my diabetes goes as far as wearing the insulin pump (with saline), to experience how it feels. My family and friends joke about Shannon being, "a wanna-be person with diabetes." He is a counselor and officer of my camp, and has helped many children to inject and to deal with negative feelings about diabetes.

I'm not saying every girlfriend or boyfriend or friend needs to become this involved in diabetes. However, I do believe it is important to feel comfortable about your diabetes around friends and to educate them about the condition. People with diabetes, as with any condition, need to be surrounded by supportive peo-ple who are knowledgeable and would be able to assist in emer-gency situations.

Many parents, although they have educated, supported, and

guided their children to take proper care of themselves, find that their child does not comply with his diabetes regimen. This is completely normal, although not healthy. Children want to be "normal." They don't want to be hassled by diabetes or by their parents concerning diabetes. Kyle, 8 years old, said, "I hate when people keep telling me to check my sugar." Children often test their parents and their diabetes to see what they can get away with. Kayla, 14 years old, agreed with Kyle, "I hate when people are constantly nagging me about my diabetes."

At the age of 12, an adolescent thinks he is invincible. Or he hopes that diabetes will go away if he ignores it. With proper education, support, and counseling, a child will understand the importance of taking care of his condition and of adhering to a regimen in order to feel good and not be sick. Your child will not understand this the first time it is explained to him. He may unfortunately need to discover this for himself. Or, with support and counseling, he may come to understand that in order to avoid getting sick he needs to take care of his condition. Continuous education is the first and most important step in allowing your child to become independent and lead a healthy life. Age-appropriate education is again the key. As your child gets older, you as a parent will become less involved in his diabetes care. Working with your diabetes health management team, and perhaps sending your child to a camp for children with diabetes, will help in making your child more responsible for and compliant with his regimen.

BUILDING RESPONSIBILITY

Your child needs to comply with his treatment regimen before he can be trusted to take on more responsibility over his treatment. (However, this should not be used as a threat because some children do not want any responsibility over their condition.) Setting goals for your child may help with his compliance. For example, one goal could be not to "sneak" food. Instead your child can discuss with you about how to cover the extra food or how to fit it into his meal plan. Once you feel comfortable that your child is not "sneaking" food and your child feels comfortable with this part of the regimen, you can move on to another goal. The next goal could be checking his sugar as prescribed by his doctor (for instance, four times a day), without putting up a fight. As these small goals are accomplished, your child is taking on more responsibility of his management.

One reason that children rebel against their parents and their diabetes regimen is that they are prohibited to eat and do certain things. If you recall your adolescence, when an adult told you not to do something, you wanted to do it even more. One of the most important things to remember is not to restrict your child because of his diabetes. If your child wants a candy bar or ice cream, allow him to have it and teach him how to fit it into his meal plan. Or teach him carbohydrate counting. If a child is allowed everything he wants to eat, he will not rebel as much and will adhere to his treatment plan better because there is no reason to sneak foods and "cheat." Think of yourself on a strict diet and remember wanting to cheat. Everyone with diabetes, including adults, will "cheat" occasionally. If you become angry with your child for "cheating" or not taking an injection, explain to him that you are concerned that he is hurting himself with this behavior. Your child will eventually learn for himself, without your having to tell him, that cheating is bad, because he will feel terrible afterwards. Your diabetes team should work with your child to find appropriate eating guidelines and accommodate insulin doses according to his eating habits and schedule. An important thing to remember is to fit diabetes into your child's lifestyle, instead of scheduling your child's life around his diabetes. Although he will still need to test his blood glucose and take injections, diabetes care can become less of a hassle.

Some children feel sorry for themselves, which is a common reaction that adults with diabetes also have. A parent's immediate response to this situation is to console the child and tell him that everything will be all right and diabetes isn't fair. You should agree with and acknowledge your child's feelings, that diabetes isn't fair and you are both angry. This form of emotional expression is good, because your child will get mad at diabetes when injection time comes around, instead of you, the parent. This behavior is appropriate for the initial shock of the diagnosis and occasionally when your child gets depressed. However, a child cannot go through life feeling sorry for himself; thinking that everything in life is ruined and having an uncaring attitude. This attitude is self-destructive. If your child's view of life is, "I have diabetes. I'm sick. What's the point of taking care of myself, I'm doomed anyway," your child may develop social problems, poor self-esteem, and health problems. Your child, and you as parent, can not sit in a "pity-pot" for the remainder of your lives. This is probably the worst thing that you can do. You need to get on with your lives and not allow diabetes to dominate or overtake it, although it does during the initial diagnosis. If you and/or your child are having problems accepting and dealing with diabetes, consider these options: seek professional help, attend support activities such as a camp, or talk with other families that have similar feelings about diabetes. I am thankful that I have a medical condition that can be controlled with medication and that I don't have a time limit to my life as more unfortunate people do. I always tell people that diabetes closed the door to my beta cells, but opened a window of opportunity. Without diabetes, I wouldn't want to become a doctor, be writing this book, or run a camp for kids.

An important lesson my parents taught me is attitude. The attitude they assumed (after they somewhat got over the initial shock), was that diabetes was not awful or anything to be ashamed of. I wasn't a "diabetic," I was still Alicia who just happens to have diabetes. A person's identity is his self-esteem, self-confidence, and attitude. I would hate my identity to be diabetes, or to be identified as a "diabetic." When a person calls me a diabetic or uses the word when referring to others, I cringe. I am not offended, but it sounds inappropriate.

I once heard a speaker addressing the topic of identity. The speaker used the following example to illustrate his point: When you are walking alone, in a strange place, with strange people, you feel uneasy. But the instant someone calls out your name, you feel more comfortable. He was emphasizing the importance of identity. Keeping this logic in mind, when someone calls me a diabetic, why would that make me feel more comfortable? Why would I want to be identified with a "disease," something that I wish I didn't have, a condition that reminds me that I am different? A person who has allergies isn't identified as an allergic, or a person who has cancer isn't "a canceric." Why would I want to be a diabetic? Why would anyone want to be identified by a chronic condition or disease after they struggle so hard to be "normal," and not to be discriminated against?

When I talk to people, I say I am a person with diabetes. It takes a little longer to say, but it doesn't sound as frightening. In my experience, people react to the word "diabetic" as if I were frail and dying. To the general public, the word "diabetic" conjures up images of a person who is going blind, or is on dialysis, or has had a foot or a few toes amputated. I think everyone with diabetes has encountered people who, after learning he has diabetes, tells him how sorry they are and how their great aunt Mary was a "diabetic" and had her foot amputated, or how their friend's father went blind because he was a "diabetic." My friend Karey, who has had diabetes for 18 years, said, "Please don't feel sorry for me. I'm very healthy and active. Diabetes is a minor part of my life." People think of a "diabetic" as a frail person who cannot lead as rigorous a life as a person who doesn't have diabetes. Telling a person that, "I have diabetes" seems less frightening. The phrase is not as threatening.

At the 1997 Circle of Life Camp kick-off, the counselors acted out a skit about a soccer game titled, "-ic's." Each character wore a large name tag that displayed his name throughout the short play. The characters were: "Normalic," "Blondic," "Hemorrhoidic," "Allergic," "Canceric," and "Diabetic." The campers thought the skit was funny, but they realized how ridiculous it sounded to call themselves "diabetics."

Children with diabetes should be identified as Susie, the best basketball player, or Johnny, the straight-A student. They should be identified with something positive, not negative. This "identity" builds a child's self-confidence and self-esteem. Having diabetes is hard enough, without constantly being reminded of it and being associated with something negative.

CHOOSING HEALTH-CARE PRACTITIONERS

An important aspect of diabetes care is your diabetes health-care team. Choosing a physician is vital for successful management of your child's diabetes. Your diabetes doctor should work with your child to design a diabetes regimen that is accommodating to your child's needs. Your child should feel comfortable with his physician, not threatened or intimated by him. Listen to your child. If he does not feel comfortable with the doctor, find a physician with whom he does feel comfortable. Ask your diabetes educator and friends about doctors. A doctor can improve your child's self-esteem and self-confidence by encouraging him and motivating him to take an active part in diabetes management.

My friend Anne, who is a nurse educator, CDE (Certified Diabetes Educator), opened her own freestanding, outpatient diabetes education facility called Diabetes Workshop, Inc., in Albany, New York. This is, in my opinion, a great learning environment for children and families. Patients are referred by doctors for one-on-one diabetes education or may be seen in a small group setting. Patients go there when they are first diagnosed; when they need to be re-educated or to brush up on some diabetes management skills; and if they are diagnosed with gestational diabetes or Type 2 diabetes. At Diabetes Workshop there is a dietitian, CDE, and a nurse, CDE who tailor diabetes education to each patient's individual needs. The environment is re-laxed and supportive. The classes are very intimate, so the per-sonal needs, concerns, and questions of the patient are adequately addressed. The teaching is done in a small room at a table, as opposed to a large room with a teacher standing in the front. Diabetes Workshop's most unique program is its adoles-cent program. When families attend classes, both the parents and child are encouraged to bring a friend or relative with them. The parents are taken into one room and the children are taught in another. A peer counselor with diabetes, a role that I have fre-quently assumed, often attends the education session with the child. The peer counselor helps teach about living with diabetes on a day-to-day basis, answering questions and concerns of the child about social issues and feelings about diabetes. The most important aspect of this program is that the diabetes education the child receives is age-appropriate, using methods and termi-nology the adolescent can understand. This type of learning en-vironment is ideal, and the health and well-being of the children improves.

A doctor should not be condescending or talk above your child's level of understanding. When your child has been edu-cated and is old enough to understand diabetes, your physician should speak directly to your child during visits, not to you about your child. The physician may talk to you about your child later. After all, your child is the patient and this gives the child a sense of responsibility over his diabetes. And if your child gets mad at diabetes, he won't be mad at you, because the doctor talked to him. Your child should feel special, involved, and trusted with information. If the trust of a physician spills over to your child's daily life, he will be more involved in his diabetes management. If children are trusted by their doctor, their diabetes team, and their parents, they are less likely to betray that trust and in turn comply with their regimen.

Your child should visit a doctor every three months. Physicians who do not specialize in diabetes may not be as informed about new treatments and information on diabetes. Research physicians in your area before choosing one. And when you find the doctor that both you and your child feel comfortable with, you and your child and the physician will grow together as a team.

Education is a continual process for your child and your family. "I learn something new every day. You always keep learning," said one parent. Other parents share that thought. "Education is never enough because every child is different in their lifestyles, treatments, growth spurts, activities, etc." As your child grows up, he will encounter different situations; his diabetes needs will change and so will his knowledge of diabetes. The doctors, nurses, and dietitians give you and your child the basic information to manage diabetes. Together, you and your child fine-tune aspects of the regimen.

Education and a positive attitude are the keys to acceptance, compliance, and assimilation of diabetes into the family, creating a supportive and understanding atmosphere. Education will build a positive attitude for your family, which will transcend to your child's emotional and social development. This integral role of education and attitude will reflect upon the physiological well-being of your child.

Chapter Summary

The best way to summarize this chapter is to quote my wise chiropractor, Dr. Diana: "To see is to know." This is what she told me during my first visit with her. I questioned her reason for taking X-rays of me, because I just wanted my back adjusted. She said that X-rays allow her to see and help educate her about my back, so that her adjustments can be more productive. This is the message I am conveying to you—educate yourself and your child. You can learn what is out there, doctors, treatments, and equipment, and then you can evaluate your needs and those of your child and determine what is appropriate. Don't be in the dark; don't put your head in the sand or follow instructions without question. You and your child are the only ones who can determine what works for your child's health and lifestyle.

Also, get a positive attitude, one that won't allow this condition to get the better of you or your child. Get an attitude of determination to get on with life. One of the best ways to attain this attitude is to hook up with families that have the same determination not only to survive, but to live long, healthy, and truly happy and fulfilled lives.

Chapter 3

Getting on with Life

PARENTS SAY...

"As a parent, it's difficult to say 'no' or explain to a 5-year-old why he can't have something his brother can."

KIDS SAY...

"When I was younger, I hated Halloween because people would give me an apple and they would give my brother candy bars."

KAREY, 21

There is no set of rules instructing parents how to deal with diabetes and raise a well-adjusted child who accepts and takes care of her condition properly. The best advice I can share with you, as a young adult who has grown up with diabetes, is to promote normalcy. What is "normal" anyway? By "normal" I mean that diabetes should not be the focus of your child's life. Yes, you should educate her, which will show her how to adjust her diabetes regimen to accommodate her lifestyle and help her learn to take care of herself. But your child should also be concerned about her upcoming basketball game, the boy who sits next her who looks like Tom Cruise, or the practical joke she played on Mike. Incorporate diabetes into normalcy. Make diabetes a lifestyle for your family instead of an enemy. The most important thing to remember is this: Incorporate diabetes into your child's lifestyle; do not incorporate her life into her diabetes regimen.

When I was first diagnosed, my parents' entire life was consumed by diabetes. Along with worries of how much a fruit exchange was, how often I could have ice cream, and how they would explain my medical condition to my family with out scaring them, their minds were filled with how will Alicia go to college, will she be able to have a baby, is she going to go blind, and will diabetes shorten her life? After dealing with the initial shock of diabetes, my parents learned how to live life one day at a time. They tried to control my diabetes together with me the best they could, in hopes of eliminating those worries of the future.

An important point to keep in mind is that you and your child live with diabetes on a day-to-day basis and know what works best for you and how your child's body reacts to different kinds of stresses. Although your physician is an expert in diabetes, everyone is different and you need to help the doctor determine what is best for your child. Diabetes management is individualized; every person is different. In order to have a healthy "normal" life with diabetes, the patient needs to work with the doctor to find an appropriate regimen. Living with diabetes is an ongoing learning process, because your food consumption, glucose levels, insulin doses, and external stresses change every day. This becomes more difficult as a child matures through puberty, because her entire body is undergoing an enormous transformation.

I was talking to a parent who expressed concern about his son's rebellious actions: not wanting to inject and sneaking food. During the course of the conversation he confessed about being too preoccupied with his son's diabetes to actually enjoy him as a kid. He explained how the week before, his son had come home from his soccer game scoring the winning goal, excited to tell his father about the game. But the first thing out of the father's mouth was, "How was your sugar during the game?" Instead of, "How did you play in the game?" As soon as the father asked about his son's diabetes, the son became angry, defensive, and hurt and screamed, "Don't you care about me and how I played? You care more about my diabetes than me!" This reaction stunned the father and he realized that, although he was concerned about his son's sugar, he should have asked later or checked on the memory of the machine later himself. This is very important. Although you are concerned about your child by asking her what her sugar is, she needs to be a kid first and get excited over other things like the goals she's achieved, and not that she has a glucose reading of 105 mg/dl (5.8 mmol/L).

It is very common to focus on the child's diabetes. It is important for parents to be actively involved and cautious about their child's diabetes, but for the psychological well-being of your child, it is of utmost importance to let your child be a "normal" kid first and talk about diabetes later. You need to look at your child as a normal kid growing up, instead of looking at her as "diabetic."

When I was 12, my best friend's family wanted to take me to Water Slide World and my mother would not let me go because of my diabetes. I was really upset. I felt as though I was being punished because I had diabetes. It wasn't fair! I told my mother that. I told her that I didn't use diabetes as an excuse, so she couldn't either. That hit a nerve with my mother, which I didn't mean to do, and she started to cry. I didn't want to hurt her, I just wanted to go to Water Slide World. I just wanted to be a kid. She kept apologizing and said she just worried about me. After that incident, I went to many functions, including class field trips and sleepovers, without much hassle over my diabetes. My parents, although they were very nervous, knew that I was able to take care of myself when I was away from home because they had educated me properly and I accepted and felt comfortable with my diabetes.

This is normalcy, being able to participate in all activities in and out of the school and enjoying myself with my friends, diabetes or no diabetes. This is very important to a child's social development. Many schools are unsure of appropriate ways to handle diabetes when certain occasions arise. If your child's school does not allow your child to participate, or they insist that you chaperone every school activity because your child has diabetes, you need to sit down and talk to the school administration. Asking your diabetes educator to do a presentation for all staff and faculty can also help. Your child should not be excluded from any school function because she has diabetes.

It is hard enough being a child with diabetes, without everyone reminding you that you are different. If your child is excluded because of her diabetes, this prejudice can have serious implications on her social, emotional, and psychological development and well-being. Many children become embarrassed or ashamed of their diabetes, thinking it is something "bad," because people who are misinformed about diabetes are prejudiced against it. Children feel that diabetes reflects on them as a person, so they take this discrimination against the condition personally. Or they become rebellious with their regimen, and they become angry at diabetes, because it prevents them from being a "normal" child. They may develop social problems, which stem from being discriminated against, because they are afraid of another rejection.

The most important thing you can do for your child is to educate the adults surrounding her, so your child is not excluded or treated differently. Also, educate your child about diabetes and the misconceptions surrounding the condition so she is prepared. If she is educated about, accepts, and feels comfortable with her diabetes, she will be able to educate her peers and adults with whom she has frequent interaction and avoid future confusions. Discriminations, prejudice, and misconceptions of diabetes and any other medical condition are caused by the lack of education. When schools, peers, and the general public are educated and understand diabetes, their misconceptions are dispelled, they are less afraid of it, and they will feel more comfortable around people with diabetes.

In addition to educating your child, instilling the proper attitude is important. Your child should know that diabetes isn't bad and it does not reflect on her persona. Diabetes is normal. Your child should believe that she is still the same person as she was before being diagnosed with diabetes. She is a person—not a "diabetic."

DIABETES AND DISCIPLINE

While counseling a couple and their child, I was astounded by the bold, almost spoiled, way the daughter was acting towards her parents. I thought, if that were my child, I would have grounded her for the next 10 years. Noticing my reaction to their daughter's lack of discipline, the parents confessed that they had been very lenient with their daughter, because they felt guilty about her diabetes. The parents told me that they were "soft on her because she is dealing with a lot more than other kids." Whether a child has diabetes or not, she needs to be disciplined. This is part of normalcy. Children may try to use diabetes as an excuse to get out of punishment or to be excused from class, but this should not be condoned. Diabetes should not be used as an excuse. You need to explain that, if they want to be a normal, average kid, they can't use diabetes as a scapegoat.

Many children do use diabetes as an excuse. I've talked with many parents who expressed concern over their child's using diabetes to be excused from class. Children need to be taught not to use diabetes as an excuse, because it could backfire and be used against them. If your child leans on diabetes as an excuse for not doing well or misbehaving, she must be taught that the condition could also be used to her disadvantage, for example, to bar her from class trips or outings with friends. This situation is difficult for you, the parents. You do not want to punish your child for having diabetes; however, you need to impress upon your child how important it is not to use diabetes as a crutch. Make an agreement with your child: she will not use diabetes as an excuse and you will not use it as an excuse against her.

Although it is very difficult for you to see your child in pain, you must be stern and insist she take her injection and check her sugar. Or if your child is old enough, insist that she perform these tasks by herself; do not allow her to depend on you. You will be hurting your child more by saying, "Just this once you don't have to take an injection." Or (if age-appropriate) "I'll do your injection just this once." Your child will feel sick later because she missed her injection or will constantly depend on you, neglecting her responsibility. Plus, allowing her to skip injections or administering injections for her, or neglecting blood-glucose monitoring when a child is young, will foster bad habits in the future. If your child gets into the habit of not doing injections, it can lead to serious problems. Explain to your child that injections, monitoring blood glucose, and following a balanced diet will make them feel good. It is very tempting for you to allow "cheating." It is also very tempting to want to do everything for your child, even if she is old enough for some independence. However, the best thing you can do for your child is to find the strength to adhere consistently to the diabetes regimen. Allow your child to vent her frustration, but insist that she follow her treatment plan. And, when she is old enough, insist that she do her own injection and blood glucose monitoring.

Although most people are not used to taking needles, living with diabetes becomes a normal lifestyle for people who have it. One parent said, "My son gets up, does his shot, eats, and our day goes on normally." Another parent said, "Living with diabetes and taking injections is as normal as brushing your teeth every day."

Parents often ask me: is it fair to punish my child by not allowing her to go out with friends because she does not check her sugar? This is difficult a question to answer because it is unfair that the child gets punished over a matter with which other children do not need to contend. However, diabetes management is vital. As a child with diabetes, I would never advise a parent to punish a child because of her diabetes management habits. It is unfair to punish a child over something that is already punishing them. If your child wants permission to sleep at a friend's house or take part in some other activity in which you will not be directly involved, talk with your child. You need to express your concern over the lack of responsibility your child has for her diabetes and the danger it poses in these situations. Your child will hopefully realize that she needs to assume responsibility over her regimen in order to have a "normal" life. This will give the child an incentive to take proper care so she is not limited by having diabetes. If you are stern with the diabetes regimen, your child will eventually understand that she cannot avoid injections, monitoring her blood glucose, or following her meal plan. And hopefully she will comply with her regimen. However, if you occasionally allow your child to neglect her diabetes care, it will be more difficult to persuade her when you want her to comply.

If your child is still resisting her diabetes regimen, even though it hinders her social life, the intervention of your doctor, diabetes educator, or a psychologist may help. Having your child attend a support group meeting or a camp for children with diabetes will also help with her compliance. Although not wanting to comply with a diabetes regimen is a typical adolescent behavior, it cannot continue unchecked for a lengthy period of time, and intervention is necessary to motivate your child to take responsibility, not only for her physiological well-being, but also for her social and psychological development. If your child misses get-togethers with friends or school functions because of her diabetes, social problems may develop in the future. The bottom line is that diabetes care is a necessity, and compliance with a diabetes regimen should begin after diagnosis to form good habits for the future.

OVERCOMING OBSTACLES

Despite your efforts and your child's efforts to lead a "normal" life, there will always be obstacles to overcome. I have learned never to use diabetes as an excuse because I never wanted it to be used as an excuse against me. I think I have always tried harder to prove that I could do anything I wanted, despite having diabetes. I never let diabetes get in the way of anything I wanted to do. And if it posed a problem, I tried even harder to make sure I attained that goal. As one parent explained, "Living a 'normal' life can happen and is definitely possible."

Since I was diagnosed with diabetes, I have wanted to become a doctor. Throughout high school I worked hard to get into a good college. I earned high honors, went to proms, and was class president, an officer for several clubs, and cheerleading captain. I worked with support groups and counseled children with diabetes, in addition to taking part in about 20 other school activities. When it was time for me to choose a college, my school guidance counselor sat me down and told me that I should look into other fields of work. She said, "The medical field is male-dominated, and with your medical condition, you'll never make it." I told her, "That's even more of a reason to go into the health care field." Well, I was determined to become a doctor and get into a medical program just to prove her wrong. When I was interviewed for the eight-year medical program that had been my dream, the interviewers concentrated on my diabetes. I thought I was being persecuted because I had diabetes. I was asked numerous questions about diabetes. One question related to my diabetes getting in the way of my schoolwork. I was so angry at this point that they hadn't asked me anything besides diabetes, I replied, "Look at my resume." But they couldn't get past my diabetes. I didn't get into the program. So I started college in a regular pre-medical program. After my first year in college, I applied to another seven-year medical program as a last resort, and I was accepted! When my guidance counselor heard, she actually apologized for insulting me. I attended that college and did very well in the program. I have now decided to become a chiropractor and attend Palmer College of Chiropractic. Your child can do *anything*. Nothing should stop her, least of all diabetes and ignorant people.

Chapter Summary

Throughout this chapter I stress the fact that parents and children should make the best of diabetes and not let it become an excuse to fail. This is easier to say than to do. I sometimes feel like I'm the person who falls off the horse and is told by everyone to get back on it if I'm ever going to learn to ride. The only thing is, most of the people telling me to get back on the horse, don't have diabetes. When I fail, I just keep trying. If you encourage your child, she will learn to push failure aside and succeed on her own terms. The sooner life goes on as it had been prior to diabetes, the better the acceptance, compliance, attitude, and long-term outcome. Once you and your child are back to your "normal" daily routine, with a few changes, of course, some days will still seem like an uphill battle. And there will be times that you and your child will feel that you just don't have time for diabetes. But together, you can overcome these changes.

Chapter 4

The Importance of Social Involvement and Support

PARENTS SAY...

"When another parent gives you advice about handling diabetes, it doesn't mean that it is right for your child. Everyone is an individual."

KIDS SAY...

"My friends are always concerned about me—if I need to eat or if I'm allowed to eat certain foods."

ASHLEY, 12

"One of the most beautiful qualities of
a true friendship is to understand and
be understood."
SENECA

"Nobody can make you feel inferior
without your consent."
ELEANOR ROOSEVELT

W hen I was first diagnosed
with diabetes, my parents wanted to send me to a diabetes camp
or bring me to a "support" group meeting for children with diabetes. I didn't want to go. I didn't have two heads. I wasn't
green. I wasn't any different from other kids, so I didn't need to
go to a "special" camp, nor did I think I needed "support."

Although I accepted my condition and was well-adjusted, or
at least I think I was, I didn't know anyone else with diabetes
besides the younger kids I was supposed to be helping. In fact,
I didn't meet anyone my age with diabetes until I was 16 and
went to the three-day American Diabetes Association's National
Youth Congress in Washington, D.C. It was awesome there!
Everyone had diabetes! If you didn't, you were a minority.
Everyone got low, checked their sugar before meals, gave insulin

injections, and had stories to share about diabetes. I felt an instant bond with people. Everyone knew about diabetes and could relate to each other in a way I never had witnessed before. I met one of my closest friends, Karey, there. Although Karey lives three states away, we talk several times a week, we vacation together, and she is a counselor at my camp. This meeting was a tremendous experience, very therapeutic. I wish I hadn't waited so long for such an experience. I now understand and appreciate the importance of diabetes camps and "support" groups, and regret not going when I was younger.

A common misconception about support activities such as camps and support groups is that everyone is sick or has problems and needs professional help. Not all support activities fit this stereotype. Most support activities for families with diabetes and other chronic conditions are composed of well-meaning and concerned individuals like yourself. These groups are composed of families struggling through the same emotions and overcoming the same obstacles. A diabetes "support" group can offer additional education for your family, as well as ideas of how to deal with certain situations your family may encounter as your child grows up with diabetes. Everyone learns from one another.

When I was first diagnosed, my doctor asked me if I would mind talking to other kids who were newly diagnosed with diabetes. I agreed, but didn't know why he would ask me to do this, because I still had two parents crying in the next room. Later he explained that I could be a role model for other kids with the condition because I accepted my diagnosis well and willingly gave myself my first injection. Unbeknownst to my doctor, I was so overwhelmed after watching my father cry, that I was too stunned to have any emotions. And the only reason I didn't object over injecting myself was that I was afraid of seeing my father cry again if I protested. I was in shock that my father, who could do anything and was the strongest person I knew, was crying and I wasn't.

That day in the doctor's office was my first introduction to counseling children and their families about diabetes and sparked my interest in becoming a doctor. Later, school nurses started asking me to talk to classes, teachers, and children with diabetes. I began a formal program that I called the "Peer Counseling and Classroom and Faculty Education Program" in the Albany Capital District Area. I visited many schools, counseled children and their families, and spoke about the psychosocial issues of diabetes at many professional events. This program was a tremendous learning experience for me. I learned something new about diabetes every time I spoke with a child who had diabetes or families of children with diabetes.

I also observed many positive changes in children with diabetes, their classmates, and school staff who received diabetes education. Misconceptions and fears were dispelled, and they felt more comfortable with diabetes. The children with diabetes felt more comfortable with and confident about their diabetes and themselves. They seemed to be less embarrassed about the condition because their classmates thought their glucose meter was "cool" and wanted to know more about it. The children started accepting their diabetes because everyone seemed interested in their condition. This supportive environment fosters acceptance of diabetes by the child with diabetes.

About six years ago I started to help with a support group for children with diabetes and their families. I took the children in one room with a certified diabetes educator to play diabetes-related games, while the parents had a roundtable discussion or listened to a speaker. The families who attended these meetings were the most understanding, strong-willed, and helpful people that I have ever met. Some parents have said to me, "I feel that there are not enough support activities in our area. I wish there were more." "There is a need for more support activities for the child with diabetes (for encouragement). Support activities in small communities are rare, but very beneficial." This group of people joined together once a month to learn new information from professionals, and to console and learn from one another, so that they could help their children. These parents realized that they had to deal with their emotions first and had to be strong in order to help their children. They empathized with one another and used each other for support. As one parent said to me, "I know I'm not alone in this struggle. Sharing my worries with other parents or helping someone is therapeutic."

The children had fun together playing games about diabetes and sharing stories about diabetes. They were very understanding when a child was upset about his diabetes or got low, or when we had a new member join our group. One parent explained, "My daughter at age 10 enjoys, and at the same time is encouraged by, these activities." This interaction was therapeutic for the children. They all looked forward to next month's meeting and our annual picnic, where they would spend all day with one another. Watching these children play together, no one would ever know that they had diabetes. They were educated about their condition, accepted it, and assimilated diabetes into their daily activities.

Local diabetes support groups are resources to explore for social interaction for both you and your child. Social interaction among parents who have children with diabetes is just as important as for the child. Parents can relate to and understand each other. Parents make a connection the same way I did with the teenagers who had diabetes. If a diabetes support group does not sound inviting, becoming involved in the Juvenile Diabetes Foundation or American Diabetes Association is an alternative way to meet people. (See Appendix 2 for a comprehensive list of local JDF chapters.) At fundraisers such as "The Walk for the Cure," which is coordinated by volunteers of the Juvenile Diabetes Foundation, you will meet people who have the same goal that you do: finding a cure for diabetes. My family and I always leave these walkathons with enough hope, excitement, and energy to move the world. Sharing experiences with other families and observing how many people support diabetes, are the most uplifting activities you can attend. Become involved in raising money, or volunteer for a diabetes charity. These organizations rely on volunteers and will welcome anyone willing to volunteer a few hours of his time. You will not be disappointed. As one parent said, "Get involved—it helps you cope."

I felt so strongly about interaction among peers with diabetes that I decided in 1996 to start my own not-for-profit camp, The Circle of Life Camp, Inc., for children and young adults with diabetes. My parents find this ironic because when I was younger, they couldn't bribe me to go to camp. If your child does go to camp and truly does not like it, or wants to be picked up early, listen to him. The camp may not be the appropriate one for him. A camper who attended my 1996 camp had attended other camps and had stayed only one night because he didn't like them. He was very apprehensive about staying at my camp. After many tears, he agreed to stay only if we agreed to call his parents if he wanted to go home. To his surprise, he had fun! When his parents came to pick him up, he cried because he didn't want camp to end. The following year he was the first registered camper for the 1997 Circle of Life Camp.

After two years of research and many adults doubting my abilities, I implemented the 1996 camp with trained counselors, an endocrinologist, a dietitian-certified diabetes educators, and nurse-certified diabetes educators. The camp was more successful than even I had hoped! The camp is held in the Adirondack Mountains on Sherman Lake. The campers and staff stay in log cabins in the woods. The camp philosophy is "fun." We promote the normalcy of living with diabetes. Campers are people with diabetes, *not* "diabetics." The campers go canoeing, swimming, hiking, play soccer, have bonfires, and do crafts, among other camping activities. Diabetes education is taught informally by counselors and nurses when questions and concerns arise. The children feel like they are at a "normal" camp. One camper said to me, "This is just like a normal camp, just like the camp my brother went to last year." At camp the children give injections, monitor their glucose together, and help one another with lows and negative feelings about diabetes. Camp motivates the children to take care of themselves. Parents have told me that they have seen tremendous results in the children after they attended camp. In some cases, children who had been hospitalized for diabetic ketoacidosis (DKA) several times the previous year, avoided the hospital the year following camp.

The Circle of Life Camp has a very relaxed, supportive and understanding atmosphere where the children feel comfortable with their diabetes and themselves. Even the apprehensive campers, who don't want to stay at first, end up exchanging addresses and making plans for next year. A strong bond forms between campers, a bond only they understand.

Children start injecting by themselves, they start checking their sugar before every meal, and talk about diabetes among other things in conversation, such as their favorite basketball teams. When children observe their peers injecting themselves, checking their sugar, and testing for ketones, a positive peer pressure occurs. Children learn that they need to take charge of their diabetes when they observe their peers taking initiative. Campers start to understand that they should join everyone else at camp and try something new, such as a new injection site or to try to adhere to their regimen. The campers are rewarded for their accomplishments at camp, which further motivates other campers to take charge of their condition, because they want to be recognized.

The words "alone" and "loneliness" are banished from my camp. Those words are as extinct as the word "diabetic." The campers form a bond with the counselors and with the other campers. The counselors do not have sympathy for these kids, but empathize with the campers. The difference between the two is like night and day; counselors should never feel sorry for the campers. This is why selecting staff is of utmost importance and should be the number one item on the priority list of any camp. The camp atmosphere is the most important aspect of camp, and staff is atmosphere. A camp may have a great location, the food may be good, and the days filled with activities; but all this pales in comparison to a great, energetic, caring, understanding, and knowledgeable staff. At the Circle of Life Camp, the chemistry between counselors and campers is instantaneous—even the parents upon meeting us for the first time said that they felt it.

The 1997 Circle of Life Camp would have been a washout (literally) if it weren't for the terrific volunteer staff. We were chilled to the bone due to uncooperative weather. If it were not for the warmth and selflessness that the highly energized counselors brought to the camp, then the children would have been bored, unmotivated about being at camp and about learning new things.

When campers leave camp at the end of the session, they should take home more than what they bring to camp. By this I don't just mean materials and tangible things. Good camps should try to provide the kids with new, updated and exciting products as well as fun stuff. However, the true and lifelong treasures the adolescents should bring home are the pride in who they are, the knowledge to equip them to manage their diabetes, the excitement in the milestones they achieved, and the confidence to gain independence. If you send your child to camp, one whose daily activities and counselors you've researched, your child will come home with something new to show you or a new perspective about diabetes and their lives. "Without the JDF and ADA fundraisers and the Circle of Life Camp the confidence and support my son has wouldn't be achieved as it is today," said one parent. At camp children cry together, laugh together, and learn together. Walls that children build to hide behind come down, and communication, acceptance, and self-confidence are built. A counselor told me last summer that she felt like she was coming home again to a wonderful, large, close-knit extended family. A young camper overheard our conversation and agreed. The camp staff and campers are all "be backers;" they all come back on their own accord.

CONVINCING YOUR CHILD

If your child is as stubborn and apprehensive as I was when I was younger, assure him that he will not be required to stay at camp if he feels uncomfortable after staying one night. Assure him that he will not be "locked in." Having strong apprehensions about attending a diabetes camp myself, I can empathize with his fears. I understand why he would not want to go to a "diabetic" camp. I'm not a "diabetic," so I didn't want to be stereotyped by going to a "special" camp. And as a child, I didn't want to spend my summer in a classroom learning about diabetes—BORING. You and your child should review information about camps together and find a camp that you both approve of. Together, you and your child should attend an open house for the camp, or meet with the staff before, to set aside fears.

As a parent, you may feel very apprehensive about leaving your child in a strange place with unfamiliar people to manage his or her diabetes. This is a huge step for parents. This is giving your child some independence from you and your control over his diabetes. Although letting go of your child is hard, this experience is beneficial for your child's psychosocial development. Camps for children with diabetes are staffed by trained counselors to accommodate your child and have health-care professionals on the premises at all times to supervise. Your child is in experienced and well-trained hands. Take these few days away from your child as a vacation from diabetes and give your needs special attention. Your child will come home excited and motivated to take care of his diabetes, and you will be refreshed to jump back into your daily routine.

The following letter exemplifies what a camp experience should be for both the child and the parent. It ties in all of the emotions prior to and after the camp in one beautiful and eloquent package:

...Rarely a day goes by that I do not think of the camp and how much it has helped our family. When [my daughter] was diagnosed seven months ago, just after her 10th birthday, we took a seat on the emotional roller-coaster that all families do when diabetes enters the lives of one they love. Now, as I look back on how far we have come and especially how incredibly well [my daughter] has done in gaining independence and a healthy approach to her diabetes, my thoughts turn to those committed to the Circle of Life Camp. My daughter was not giving her own injections when she left for camp, but quickly learned at camp, and does almost every one now. Her attitude is positive and her confidence has flourished. She speaks of camp often—of going next year and the year after!

Chapter Summary

No man is an island, as they say; we all need to belong, to be "cool," to be "in." What all this means is that we only want to be accepted into society and the human race in the least painful way possible. We don't want to blend in, but in some way to complement the human decor. No one wants to be perceived as weak or a misfit. Society depicts people, cars, houses, and lawns as flawless or perfect. If any of the above are blemished or flawed in any way, they are immediately recalled or looked down upon. In other words, the are not "in," "cool," or sought after by any means.

Having diabetes makes a child feel like a misfit. I often thought of myself as one of the misfit toys in the Christmas cartoon "Rudolph the Red Nosed Reindeer" whenever my parents mentioned a camp or diabetes support group. I felt I was being banished to some island with the other misfits. Now I own one of these camps because I came to realize, after volunteering at support groups and camps, that the children who attended these social activities were the most intelligent, loving, and understanding people I had ever met, and I was actually one of them. These children have a vocabulary of a medical student and could go one-on-one with the best of them. These young people have courage. They could face multiple needles a day. (I wouldn't even want to calculate how many per year that would be.) This kind of bravery is very hard to find. Many linebackers have fainted at the mere mention or sight of just one needle, let alone a trash bag full. The compassion these children show one another is remarkable; they openly welcome a newcomer in "misfit" land and share their feelings. Personally, I feel that we all belong, that we are a whole, and together we can handle anything life throws our way.

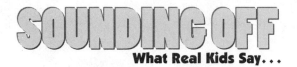

SOUNDING OFF
What Real Kids Say...

"I find it hard to go to a party and re-member to take my insulin or let people know that I have diabetes."

COREY, 16

Chapter 5

Working Through Frustrations

PARENTS SAY...

"I believe that my son's independence began when he started doing his own shots."

KIDS SAY...

"My advice to parents is not to be overprotective and crowd your child. Give them some freedom to grow."

CORI, 16

"Experience is not what happens to man; it is what man does with what happens to him."
ALDOUS HUXLEY

"Finish every day and be done with it. You have done what you could; some blunders and some absurdities crept in—forget about them as soon as you can. Tomorrow is another day!"
RALPH WALDO EMERSON

Diabetes is a continuous balancing act. Adjusting insulin according to a glucose reading, checking blood sugar, eating the appropriate foods at the right time, exercising, carrying food at all times, and so on. This balancing act does get frustrating. There are times when, no matter what we do, our sugar is high. Or, we get low at the most inopportune times—like when we are giving an oral report in front of the class. It happens to everyone, no matter how long they have had diabetes. No one is perfect. We do the best we can do.

As a parent you get upset when your child's glucose is high, even though you and your child followed the doctor's instructions exactly. This is very aggravating and discouraging. Children are growing and their hormones are on overdrive. They are exploring and learning new things. They get angry and nervous.

This all affects your child's glucose level. It is hard to accept that your child is not going to have absolutely perfect glucose control, and her sugar will not always read 105 mg/dl (5.8 mmol/L) on the meter. She will have high glucose readings occasionally and sometimes more than occasionally. Some days I will do everything I am supposed to do and I have a glucose reading of 278 mg/dl (15.4 mmol/L). My mother asks me why and I answer, "I have diabetes." I'm not trying to be facetious, but it's a fact. Some things you just don't have control over, such as getting nervous about a test and two hours later your sugar is 300 mg/dl (16.7 mmol/L).

I was at the ocean this past summer watching the calm body of water, which had only a few ripples to disrupt its peaceful rhythmic flow. The tranquil state of the water and the serene atmosphere lasted for an hour. I wished I could sit on the beach forever. But I couldn't. The wind picked up and the calm water was disturbed by the growing waves. My tranquil state was beginning to change into one of anxiousness, as the wind began to blow more and more. I began to feel frustrated at the sand in my face and my hair blinding my sight.

The ocean is like our bodies when diabetes blows into our lives. Diabetes disturbs the balance of nature with its highs and lows, which we do not have any control over. Diabetes takes over without warning, without thought or regard for that wonderful balance and calm, tranquil state that the rest live in. But, we do as I did at the ocean—pick ourselves up, and struggle to gain control. We hope that tomorrow the calm seas, the days of normal glucose readings, will outnumber the frustrating ones.

I was listening to a speaker talk about the kaleidoscope of

emotions that accompany diabetes. At a support group meeting for children with diabetes and their parents, the speaker asked the families to finish the following sentence: Diabetes is____. Some of the responses were: scary, frustrating, hopeful, challenging, a lifestyle, and depressing. The following month the families were asked the same question, and most of them gave different answers than they had the previous month. Families who had said diabetes was hopeful the month before said it had become frustrating the following month, or vice-versa. Dealing with diabetes on a daily basis becomes a roller coaster ride of emotions. You have some bad days and you have goods days. Everyone does, parents and children included.

Diabetes becomes frustrating to children. They want to forget they have it. They rebel, not taking injections or sneaking three candy bars before they get home from school. Sometimes they become angry at anyone who mentions diabetes. Moira, age 11, says, "I hate being forced to eat (when I'm low)." This is normal, just like any other feelings you or your child has about diabetes. Listen to and acknowledge your child's feelings about diabetes. Acknowledging your child's feelings and allowing her to get angry at diabetes may help her accept her treatment plan. Everyone with diabetes gets tired of the yo-yo of sugar readings and adhering to their regimen. If you have ever tried a "fad" diet, you know how hard it is to keep to a regimen. A friend said, "I am about to rip this insulin pump out! I feel like a yo-yo—I'm 40 mg/dl one minute and 400 mg/dl the next!! And I feel as if a 18-wheeler just ran over me!"

Having diabetes is frustrating because it greatly affects the way you feel physically. Kimberly, age 9, says, "I hate ketones."

The week before my SAT I took extra care of myself to ensure that my sugar would be "normal" and I would feel good for the test. An hour before the test, my sugar was 140 mg/dl (7.8 mmol/L). I was prepared; I brought water if I got thirsty and food if I got low. Well, before the test I became very thirsty and drank *a lot* of water. In the middle of this timed test I used the restroom a few times, and by the end, I was nauseous and got sick two times. My sugar was over 450 mg/dl (25 mmol/L). I was talking to a teacher about what happened during the test and she said, "You should have taken better care of yourself." As if it was my fault that I got nervous and purposely made my sugar high!

Another frustration of mine when I was growing up: I hated and I still hate when people without diabetes talk to me condescendingly about how I should be controlling my diabetes. I understand that doctors and nurses have gone to school for many years to become educated about diabetes and other people giving me guidance and advice are well meaning. However, if a person doesn't have diabetes, she shouldn't act as if everything is so easy! The most educated and understanding people have tried to simulate life with diabetes by giving multiple injections, wearing the insulin pump, or counting carbohydrates. I find it difficult to understand how a health professional can tell you what you are supposed to be doing and act as if it's easy, if they haven't tried it. Diabetes would be easy if you gave yourself three injections a day and your sugar was always 100 mg/dl (5.6 mmol/L) or even if your sugar did bounce up and down, but you never felt ill. But there are hundreds of other factors that need to be included besides medicine. When I went on the insulin pump, I was instructed to put the pump under my pillow at night to keep it out of my way. The first night I couldn't sleep, because the pump I wear makes a clicking sound every time it delivers one-tenth of a unit of insulin (I get 1.5 units of insulin per hour). The next morning I told the nurse that I wanted her to try putting the pump under her pillow. She did not realize that it had such a loud clicking sound!! My advice to parents and health professionals: before you instruct your child/patient to do something, try it yourself.

When I was younger and my sugar was low, I could eat the entire contents of our refrigerator. When your adrenaline is pumping, you feel like you're passing out and you know that eating will make you feel better. It's hard to control how much you eat. You want to eat until you feel better, which takes at least fifteen minutes. I hated when my mother said, "Give the food a chance to work; you don't need to eat that much." At that point, when I'm low and shaky, I would eat my mother's head to get my sugar up, forget about the extra cookies or juice. I'm in a panic! Give me food! My friend who also has diabetes and I joke about nighttime hypoglycemia. We agree that when you get low in the middle of the night, you inhale half of the refrigerator and the next morning your parents can't make breakfast because you've eaten all the food. Ron, 14 years old, agrees: "I hate waking up at 2 a.m. and being low."

I'll never forget when I stopped into the mall to look at a shirt and I didn't bring any food or money with me. I got a severe hypoglycemic reaction. I was in a panic; I didn't know what to do. I wanted to call my parents, but they couldn't do anything from home and they would be very upset that I was not equipped to deal with it. I went to three restaurants and finally an ice cream shop gave me a regular soda because I looked pale. I was so embarrassed. I learned my lesson, though, and I have never left home without my meter or glucose tablets again. This situation is one of the most common frustrations among parents—worrying. One parent explained, "My frustration is worrying about him and allowing him to go wherever he wanted. I didn't like letting go of him, but I had to. It was a big adjustment for me rather than him."

During my junior year in high school I worked in a clothing store in the largest mall in New York State. Everyone knew I had diabetes and that I kept food behind the counter in case I felt low. I worked long hours on my feet as well as exercising daily. I guess I put too much strain on my feet and my arches collapsed. I was in a lot of pain, but didn't tell anyone. I went in the back room to check my sugar because I felt faint. My glucose reading was 125 mg/dl (6.9 mmol/L), so I wasn't low. But I felt like I was going to pass out. I was walking out of the back room and fell. The next thing I knew, the ambulance was there and three EMT's were trying to hook me up to a glucose IV and take my insulin pump off me. I kept protesting because I wasn't low and I needed my insulin pump. Everyone thought I had passed out because of my diabetes, but I really fainted because of my feet hurt so much. By the time I got to the hospital, my sugar was 450 mg/dl (25 mmol/L) and they needed to start an insulin drip! Luckily I was only in the hospital for two hours, but I did need to quit my job.

Diabetes is also frustrating because people your child will encounter may have a distorted view of the condition, which leads to uncomfortable or embarrassing situations. If your child is educated about diabetes, she will be able to deal with these situations appropriately. During my first year in college I had asked one of the cafeteria cooks if the Jell-O was sugar-free, because I needed to know how much carbohydrate was in the Jell-O (I wear an insulin pump and carbohydrate count). On the way out of the cafeteria, I grabbed some candy and brought it to the cashier, who overheard my conversation with the cook. In the middle of the cafeteria the cashier loudly protested my purchase of candy. She told me that I couldn't have candy because I had diabetes. She informed me that her aunt had diabetes for 20 years and had had her foot amputated because she ate too much candy. She said to me, "I will not stand by and let you kill yourself by eating sugar." I was completely embarrassed with the entire cafeteria now looking at me. I tried to explain to her that things are different than they were 20 years ago and people with diabetes can have candy now. She allowed me to buy the candy, but that incident cured my sweet tooth for quite a while.

Sometimes I feel like I'm in a comic strip and diabetes is the main character. As I mentioned, I wear an insulin pump. The pump is about the size of a deck of cards and is attached to a tube connected to a small canula, which is inserted under the skin in the abdomen. I can't feel anything in my stomach and hardly realize that I'm attached to something. The pump is a challenge for women to wear sometimes, though. Wearing the pump with certain clothing is like a game! Where should I put the pump when I wear a dress? I usually wear the pump in my stocking against my thigh, to conceal it when I wear a skirt above the knee. This is where I put my pump when I went to a meeting with school officials. I was an officer on the college student senate, acting as a representative of the student body at this particular meeting with the college vice president, dean, and other important officials. The meeting was closing and suddenly my pump alarm started to ring. Everyone looked around for the beeping sound. The restroom was occupied, so I could not shut the pump off because it was in my pantyhose. It continued to beep every three minutes for the rest of the meeting, but everyone was too polite to ask why there was noise coming from in between my legs, and I was too embarrassed to explain.

I was stopped by airport security when I went to Sweden, because the batteries inside my pump set off the metal detector alarm. Looking back on the event I can laugh, but at the time, when the Swedish-speaking police tried to take the insulin pump away from me because they thought it was a bomb, I was scared. I had a difficult time explaining to them that the pump was medical equipment. You should have seen their reaction when I showed them it was attached to my stomach!

SOLVING FOOD ISSUES

One of the most frustrating things for parents is food. Diabetes wouldn't be as worrisome and frustrating for parents if food didn't play such an influential role in diabetes management. The most frequently asked question is, "How can I get my child to eat what she is supposed to?" My answer is education for both your and you child. One parent's advice is, "Try to keep an open mind. Flexibility is the key." The most important thing is not to deprive them of food such as ice cream, candy, and cookies. Remember: A person with diabetes can eat *anything* and *everything* a person without diabetes can eat. A person with diabetes just needs to adjust her insulin and/or fit the food into her meal plan. A "diabetes diet" is a healthy diet, a diet everyone should follow.

Carbohydrate counting allows a person with diabetes to choose what food she wants to eat, based on the carbohydrate content in the food. Everything you eat has carbohydrate in it, except for protein and fat. Food servings of milk, breads/starches, and fruit have 15 grams of carbohydrate in them. For example, a piece of bread, 1 cup of milk, and a small apple all have 15 grams of carbohydrate. A serving of vegetables has 5 grams of carbohydrate. A sample lunch of 60 grams of carbohydrate for your child could be: 1 ham sandwich, a glass of milk, and a small apple; 1 cup of spaghetti, a glass of milk, and 1/2 cup canned peaches. They can pick and choose what food they want to eat, which will hopefully discourage them from "sneaking" foods. Your child should eat a healthy diet, just as a child without diabetes should. You should work with your dietitian for a meal plan that can accommodate your child's lifestyle and age.

A tip for parents is not to constantly scold or nag your child about her "diet." We know you are worried about our blood sugar getting too high. You're also concerned about it going to low. My parents said they felt helpless and fearful because they did not know how I felt when I was low and shaky, or when I was high and had cotton mouth. My parents always wanted to know how I felt when I was low—you panic! Everyone has different symptoms of hypoglycemia and they may change during the course of your child's life. Have your child explain to you how they feel, so that you are aware of her visible symptoms of hypoglycemia. When your child is low, act fast! Hypoglycemia is a terrible feeling.

Raising your voice or constantly nagging about what your child "should" or "shouldn't" eat goes in one ear and out the other, or it may cause her to cheat more often out of spite. Many kids at my camp agreed with Ron, age 14, when he expressed his frustration about constantly being nagged: "It gets annoying." They hate diabetes and by yelling and nagging you are pushing them to hate it more. Nathan, age 14, said, "One of the most frustrating things, one of the things I hate most about diabetes, is checking my blood sugar frequently and being reminded to do it." Kristen, age 12, and Daniel, age 10, agree that "taking extra shots to cover for highs is annoying." By shouting at your child you show them your lack of control and frustration at diabetes. You are actually shouting at the diabetes, not your child. And, in turn, no one has control, and diabetes ends up winning. Make diabetes into something livable, and you may have an occasional high reading because your child ate too much cake, but it is worth the sacrifice by avoiding World War III. Becky, age 11, says that her biggest complaint is, "not being able to eat what your friends are eating."

With all the emphasis on food, it's not surprising that eating disorders are a very real problem for many people with diabetes, especially young women. To some, food becomes an enemy— especially when they're trying to lose weight, or are not hungry. Some either refuse to eat in order to stay thin or eat normal amounts but then purge the food by inducing vomiting or taking laxatives. Others find that they can control their weight by intentionally reducing or omitting insulin doses, thereby spilling ketones in the urine. If you notice that your daughter or son is unusually preoccupied with food or weight, seek professional help. Eating disorders are serious. They can affect a person's diabetes control, physical development, and mental well-being.

DIABETES AND PUBERTY

As your child goes through puberty she experiences a variety of changes and that affect her diabetes needs. During puberty your child will eat more because she is growing, so it is important to visit your dietitian to insure that your child is receiving the appropriate caloric intake. Your child may also need to adjust her insulin frequently because of hormonal changes within her body. Although your child may be doing her best to comply with her regimen and adjustments the doctor makes, her glucose readings may not show it. This causes a feeling of hopelessness and frustration for your child. Be understanding and encouraging. Trying to adhere to a regimen and not achieving the expected results is very disappointing and discouraging. Your child may have the attitude, "What difference does it make what I do?" Reassure your child that this is a temporary change she is going through. Share your child's disappointment and reward her for her efforts.

There is no vacation from diabetes. There are no breaks. We must constantly take injections, have highs and lows, and plan ahead to incorporate diabetes into our day—every day. One parent explained, "Summer vacation is very frustrating because my daughter feels that she's on vacation and should be able to sleep in and eat what and when she wants. But, she can't. Because of diabetes she has to get up at a certain time for insulin and breakfast." This is sometimes discouraging because we work very hard

79

to adhere to our doctors orders with the goal of achieving "near-normal" blood glucose readings. Although our goal is to have normal HbA1c's to avoid complications, there is no prize at the end of a child's hard work, such as diabetes going away. When you are on a weight-loss program, although your efforts seem tireless and you sometimes get discouraged, you have a specific goal—say, to lose 20 pounds. And when you do lose the weight your goal is achieved. There is a change in your life—new clothes sizes and people complimenting you on your figure. With diabetes, although the goal of constant normal blood-glucose reading is a phenomenal accomplishment, children get discouraged because there is no visible difference in their lives (besides feeling good). They still need to do injections, watch what they eat, etc. Rewarding your child for her tireless efforts is important.

Children become very discouraged when, although they have done everything in their power to keep their sugar down, they are high. Children feel very guilty about this, although it is sometimes no fault of their own. As long as your child's glucose readings are high through no intentional cause, treat them casually. Troubleshoot together with your child to see if there was something that might have contributed. This does not necessarily mean anything that they consumed. High blood-glucose readings could be caused by hormones during puberty or environmental stressors. Talk with your child about her day or week. It may be insignificant to parents, but a bad hair day, a blemish, or not being picked for the team in gym class can devastate and panic an adolescent. This in turn can make blood glucose soar; in some people it causes hypoglycemia or it may not affect your child at all. But taking that burden off her shoulders and talking about a problem can decrease her stress level. Absolving your child of any wrongdoing in regards to her diabetes can also help her lower her stress level. Seeing a high sugar reading and feeling guilty will also contribute to an even higher glucose reading and can further increase her emotional stress level. Work together with your child to absolve her of guilty feelings over her glucose readings.

As your child grows up into adulthood, the blemishes turn into wrinkles and the bad hair day turns into a job interview or bill payments. Being able to recall how to deal with stress from her childhood will help her deal with her current stressors and will help keep her calm. The more positive experiences your child has dealing with stressful situations, the better prepared she will be for future crises.

Diabetes requires a continuous learning process throughout life. Diabetes and the treatment of the condition are very individualized. This is what makes diabetes so difficult to manage. For example, when I am upset about something, my blood sugar can fly up to 350 mg/dl (19.4 mmol/L) within an hour; whereas a camper of mine told me whenever he gets nervous, he gets low. Doctors, nurses, dietitians, and books can give you suggestions and ideas of how to deal with diabetes, but it is up to you and your child to figure out what works best. This also can be very challenging. To figure out what works for your child, you may need to experiment. For example, whenever I eat bologna for lunch, I get unexplained high sugar readings at night. This is probably due to the high fat content in the processed meat.

An evident factor that exemplifies diabetes variability from person to person is the amount of insulin a person takes and in which combinations. When I was in my early teens, I took three times the amount of insulin than a man twice my weight ordinarily would. These unique requirements for each person become very frustrating, because there are no absolute generalizations of how to manage diabetes, aside from the fact that we need to take insulin and eat when we are low. And when you finally think that you have figured out how to manage your child's diabetes, she hits puberty and you enter a whole new ball-game.

Chapter Summary

I have mentioned once before that I do not have time for diabetes; my life is far too busy and I have many things to accomplish. Stopping and eating, checking my sugar, or injecting just get in my way, as I'm sure it does for you and your child. The lows and highs during soccer games, piano lessons, cheerleading, during a test, or just hanging out with friends is just plain *frustrating*.

The next best thing to a cure for me would be to inject and not worry if I will get low or become high, so that I could lead a more predictable lifestyle. We are in the same boat, and though it is not sinking, it is a bit too rocky for me, as it probably is for you. The person who said, "Laughter is the best medicine" must have had diabetes. There are days that I know if I don't laugh, I will most surely cry. The jugglers in the circus have nothing on people with diabetes. The juggling of food, insulin, glucose monitoring, highs, lows, and the most fun—ketones—before a test, a prom, a date, a sleepover, or sometimes before breakfast is impressive. So we try to fix what is wrong, eating if we're low, injecting if we are high (so what's a little needle prick if it helps us continue with our day?). When one of my friends complains about her day—her hair wouldn't comb right, she found a blemish somewhere, or she had to take a big test—I smile to myself and think, my day was great: I controlled an acne breakout, tamed my unruly mane, took a test, and saved my life, too!

Chapter 6

A Declaration of Independence

PARENTS SAY...

"Letting go and allowing my daughter to become independent was the hardest thing for me to do. As I watched her do things for herself, it was very tempting to take over."

KIDS SAY...

"My parents are overprotective of me, but I know it because they are concerned."

NATHAN, 13

"I believe that anyone can conquer
fear by doing the things he fears to do
provided he keeps doing them until he
gets a record of positive experiences
behind him."
ELEANOR ROOSEVELT

I ndependence means different
things to different people. Being on one's own; making major as
well as minor decisions; not being in a dependent state. These are
all examples of independence. For all to factor in, you must
be educated, informally guided, and nurtured by another independent person. This also brings up another question: How independent are we, anyway? We all in some way depend on
something or someone. Independence may also mean confidence
in one's own judgment and competence—no matter who depends on us or we on them. We all must make that distinction on
our own. That's what independence is—if only we were confident enough to do that.

I once asked my parents when and how long it took for them
to wean me off their dependence. They said that they were won-

dering the same thing, only in reverse. That is, when will my mother and my father wean themselves from me,and their dependence on me. That certainly made me stop and think. Parents depend on their children for their sanity and their love, even though we drive them insane at times. But my mother said that kids keep parents stabilized and grounded, just as much as parents instill security in kids. If one has a gift and no one to give it to, what good is it? Love is the gift that both parties receive. Love is given freely to one another, no matter what, no matter when. Love is given to each other independently.

At the Circle of Life Camp, kids come to camp and become part of a whole, yet remain quite independent. Everyone at camp has diabetes, so the children feel like they belong; they become part of this group. Independence is well stressed and encouraged by informal education. Confidence is instilled by allowing the children to become actively involved in their diabetes, by discussing their insulin dosages and coverage scales as well as other aspects and concerns about their regimen. Having an active role in their diabetes care motivates the campers to assume responsibility for their diabetes regimen.

Another band in the independence spectrum, which is the ultimate goal of parents and children, is to have parents forget about their child's diabetes. Could you ever believe that you could forget even for a moment, an hour, better yet—a whole day! Diabetes is always there, forever etched in their minds and hearts. But try to look at your child as a whole without mentioning the words, "diabetes," "sugar readings," "high," "low," or "injections." Be with your child and don't mention anything related to diabetes for that day, party, or even a weekend.

Do you know what this would mean? Do you know what a phenomenal accomplishment this would be for you and your child? This is true independence—the independence of mind, body, and soul. Independence breeds wonderful, deep trust between people. The final absolution, the baptism of no guilt; no "what ifs;" just the "now."

My mother has strange little sayings that she has heard along the way. One of them is, "How does one eat an elephant?" ... "One bite at a time." There is truth in this saying. A person's goals are achieved one day, one step, one trust at time. That is how your child assumes responsibility and eventually independence with his diabetes.

LETTING GO

Independence is a topic that produces a lot of anxiety among parents. "It is tough to let go. Children need to make choices, both right and wrong, and we as parents hope they learn from their mistakes," said one parent. All parents fear for their child's safety and well-being. Diabetes complicates the "growing up" process. Not only do parents worry about their child's personal safety at public places when they are not present to supervise, but also if they have food with them in case they get low, extra insulin, or if they will check their sugar before activity to prevent hypoglycemia or ketoacidosis. Nathan, age 14 said, "My parents are very nervous. They never let me stay overnight at my friend's house." Parents worry if their child will know what to do in the event they are low or if someone else knows what to do in the event of an emergency. Parents are nervous when they allow their child to sleep at a friend's house. Parents are afraid to lose control over their child's diabetes. A parent of an 11-year old girl said to me, "I feel that as long as I'm her mother and I am there for her, I'll give her insulin and feed her as she needs. When she's spending the night at a friend's house, she does fine taking care of her diabetes—I know she can if she has to."

Another parent shares her wisdom: "Parents need to loosen their grip. When children are young, parents need to give them choices—both good, but different so the child can feel confident." Responsibility over diabetes should begin when children are first diagnosed or when they reach an age when they have the cognitive skills to make choices and help, even in small ways, with their management. As your child matures, he should be given age-appropriate information about diabetes. As you continue to educate your child, you should encourage him to take gradual responsibility over his diabetes management. For example, a 5-year-old boy I used to baby-sit could push the button on the lancet device to prick his finger and push down the plunger after his parents injected him.

Some children are anxious to gain responsibility over their diabetes management. Cori, age 15 said, "Let us take over, give us more independence." Others want to forget that they have the condition, and prefer that their parents take care of it. In both scenarios, education is the bottom line. Education is the key to acceptance, self-confidence, and independence. If your child wants to take charge of his diabetes care, education will provide the foundation for success. If your child is still hesitant, education will hopefully motivate him to take care of himself.

Independence is not a black-and-white issue. Just as a child learns gradually to walk and talk, a child will gradually learn to assume responsibility over his treatment regimen. A child needs to be supported, encouraged, and rewarded for his milestone accomplishments. An accomplishment may be checking his glucose before every meal or taking the initiative to check for ketones when his sugar is 300 mg/dl (16.7 mmol/L) or explaining to his friends about diabetes. Every positive step toward accepting diabetes and accepting some responsibility over the condition is a huge achievement. Growing up with pressure from peers and stereotypes is difficult, and every step toward overcoming the obstacle of diabetes should be recognized.

At my camp, when a camper tries something new such as injecting into a new site, injecting for the first time, mixing his own insulin, checking for ketones without being told, or showing even a small improvement in his diabetes care or attitude, he is recognized for his personal achievement. At each meal the children are recognized and applauded by the rest of camp for their achievement, and the campers also get to choose a prize from the prize box. This instills pride and motivates the children to improve their diabetes-management skills. This confidence and responsibility fosters independence and acceptance of their condition. The children leave camp feeling confident with themselves and their diabetes.

Becky, 11 years old, said, "My mother always wants to know why my sugar is high and wants to help with my injection. But I can do this by myself!" Although parents want their child to be educated and proficient in diabetes management, they are used to controlling every aspect of their child's life. And when they are not actively involved in a part of their child's life, they begin to panic. As a parent, you need to trust that you have equipped your child with the knowledge, skills, and self-confidence to manage his diabetes and handle any situation that may arise.

A parent of a 14-year-old boy suggested, "My advice is to know where he is; who he is with; and someone who knows what to do if his blood glucose gets too low. A check-in point somewhere in the day is great and has worked out well." As your child matures, he will want more privacy and to make more decisions on his own.

BUILDING TRUST

You need to form a trust with your child. You need to explain to him that, before he is allowed some independence, he needs to show some trust and responsibility. For example, many parents have told me that their children refuse to follow a meal plan and sneak candy after school when they are alone. Explain to your child that there should be no reason to "sneak" food, because he can fit foods in his meal-plans or take extra insulin to accommodate the extra carbohydrate.

In order for your child to learn how to fit certain foods into his diet, make an appointment with a dietitian. Allow the dietitian to talk with your child and figure appropriate guidelines for a flexible diet. If a medical professional discusses directly with your child appropriate ways to manage diabetes, it takes the burden off you. And if your child becomes frustrated with his diabetes, the "blame" for their diabetes regimen is off of you, the parents. By "blame," I mean that the child's angry frustrations about being "made" to take injections or check for ketones will be less likely directed toward you, the parent, and more at the diabetes. Although this seems like an insignificant thing at first, it alleviates guilty feelings. When a child gets angry, he is less likely to say, "You make me do injections" or "You won't let me eat that extra piece of cake," because the doctor or nurse told them. Although children do not intend to make their parents feel guilty about taking injections, their angry frustrations upset parents at a deep level.

Sometimes independence becomes a tug of war with parents and children. You are naturally overprotective of your children. You also do not want to give your child enough rope to hang himself. But there is a time when children need to be trusted and given support to manage their diabetes by themselves in order to grow up socially and psychologically well acclimated. For example, at the age of 15, a teenager should be able to go to a sleepover party without his parents coming to give him an injection or calling his parents before he eats something.

Ideally, independence is a natural progression for you and your child. But many times independence becomes a difficult issue—either the child wants to assume more responsibility than you are ready to give; or the child wants to stay dependent on his parents, neglecting responsibility as a form of denial or anger. If your child is ready to take responsibility over his diabetes management and is well educated, allow him more responsibility slowly.

When your child is confident and appropriately carries out his responsibilities, allow him more independence. Try to incorporate diabetes responsibilities with independence in everyday activities. For example, if your child maintains his responsibility of checking his sugar before every meal, allow him to go to the mall with friends and have lunch. There is no set age at which children are ready for certain responsibilities. You need to assess your child's understanding, maturity, and capabilities with your child's doctor to determine the level of responsibility your child should have over his regimen. You determine your child's level of responsibility over his diabetes, just as you do in daily activities such as going to the mall with friends. Your child should feel comfortable with what he is doing. For example, I have met kids 10 years old who could handle their diabetes regimen by themselves if allowed, but I have also met 15-year-old adolescents who still need to depend on their parents to tell them how much insulin they should take.

Allowing your child to have independence over his regimen is not a final or ending communication with you over his diabetes. He should and will ask for your advice or discuss how he should do something. And you can occasionally ask him his sugar readings or look at the meter yourself, to see how he is managing. Allowing your child to have independence from you in managing his regimen is a natural process that is beneficial to both you and your child. It is something that you both can feel good about. As one parent explained, "Knowing that my main purpose is to prepare my child for adulthood, we discuss her care together, and she is learning to make her own decisions. With each success she gains more confidence. This makes me feel positive about her growing independence."

Parents need to educate, support, and encourage their child to make decisions on his own. During early adolescence a decision could be to take a shot in the arm or in the stomach. As the child approaches his teens, he will learn and make decisions about appropriate food choices and substitutes, as well as how much insulin to give himself with the guidance of his parents. I stress guidance because you want control and when your child does not make the same choice that you would, you take over, and that can take away from your child's self-confidence. Liam, age 20, advises parents: "Adolescents do not want to be told what to do by their parents; they want suggestions." When your child makes a decision, as long as it will not harm him or produce huge negative effects, support him in his decision. If your child makes a poor choice and does not like the result, he will learn for next time. And if his choice results in a positive experience, then your child teaches you something.

When your child makes unwise choices, such as skipping an injection or eating candy bars without covering, you need to discuss with him in a mature fashion what occurred, why, and how to prevent that incident in the future. Although your immediate response may be to yell and disapprove of your child's decision by punishing him, this does not improve your child's judgment in making decisions. If this type of behavior is intentional and repetitive, you may need to offer more suggestions when your child is making decisions or take him to a nurse educator who will re-educate him and help solve some problems he may have managing his diabetes.

If your child is very dependent on you for his diabetes care and you feel he should assume more responsibility, talk to him and try to figure out why he does not want to take some initiative. Your diabetes educators and doctor can help. Your child may need to be re-educated and attend some activities where there are other children with diabetes.

It is very common for young teenagers to want to be popular

and be "cool." Diabetes isn't "cool" so teens try to avoid it as much as humanly possible by eating whenever they want, not checking their sugar, not checking for ketones, or skipping injections because they don't want their friends to see them doing something "uncool." The first step to turning diabetes from something "uncool" to something "normal" (it doesn't need to be cool to live with it) is accepting the condition. Your child needs to accept that he has diabetes whether he wants it or not.

Accepting diabetes is vital for children as well as parents in order to manage diabetes. You can set an example by accepting diabetes. Your child may need professional counseling, which is very common, or he may need to be re-educated to understand diabetes in its entirety. Camps and support groups for children foster acceptance because diabetes is the norm there. When a teenager realizes that he is not alone and not "different," then he will begin to accept diabetes as a normal part of his life. Meeting with and talking to others with diabetes helps this process. Accepting diabetes and becoming comfortable with yourself and the condition is gradual. This process should start at diagnosis, so that when your child matures and takes on more responsibility becoming independent, this will be a natural process, a natural progression that both you and your child feel comfortable with.

Once a child accepts diabetes and is not ashamed or embarrassed by it, he will be able to make better decisions regarding management. When a child accepts his diabetes and is educated about it, he will hopefully feel comfortable enough to tell his friends. The embarrassment of going to the restroom to take an injection will diminish. Diabetes becomes a part of everyday life, and decisions of how much insulin he should take or what he should eat becomes automatic.

My sister Alaina becomes annoyed when someone asks about her future plans and aspirations. At 17, she's wise beyond her years. My sister's philosophy is "People are forever looking for tomorrow, and forget to enjoy and savor the now and today." Diabetes throws a curve ball into a person's life, throwing him off balance. A person needs to feel comfortable and regain his center of gravity with his current situation before he can move on. A person needs to feel grounded and confident with himself before moving on to the next stage of life.

Diabetes is truly an unpleasant, intrusive, and frustrating lifestyle. But if you make the best of it, it can help form a bond between you and your child. Amazingly enough, something so seemingly awful at first may be the very thing that helps us count our blessings. You and your child can learn together. The key here is learning together; not one teaching and preaching to the other, but listening. Living with and learning about diabetes is like growing up together, learning to live life happily, healthfully and to its fullest potential. This super-glue of love, trust, and growing will never let parents and their children down.

Chapter Summary

This chapter is a form of self-healing, an answer to a call for help in the search for chronic dependence. As a child grows up and matures, the need for independence becomes more apparent. Even a baby takes its first steps away from his parents and toward what used to be the unattainable: the doorway or another person in the room. Teenagers dream of their driver's license and being out on the open road. This sounds disastrous to parents because you fear for the worst, yet you bite the bullet and teach your child how to drive and instill safe rules and regulations.

So then, you, as a parent, must do the same for your child with diabetes. You must put him behind that syringe and teach him to navigate good habits for good health. After all the nurturing, loving, and years of right and wrong, you must eventually feel confident enough to send your child out on his independent journey, with you not too far behind. The excitement a person feels from, "I can do it myself" far exceeds any other. This satisfaction can lead to many other accomplishments as well. The pleasure that you will both feel in each other's trust will lead to a strong and everlasting love.

SOUNDING OFF

What Real Kids Say...

"You know who your real friends are—the people who watch out for you, asking if you need anything to eat or if you're allowed to have that."

KAREY, 21

Diabetes Organizations and Resources

American Association of Diabetes Educators (AADE)—To find a diabetes educator in your area
444 North Michigan Ave., Suite 1240
Chicago, IL 60611
(800) TEAMUP4

Juvenile Diabetes Foundation International (JDF)—For information on upcoming JDF events. (See Appendix 2 for addresses and phone numbers of local chapters.)
120 Wall St., 19th Floor
New York, NY 10005–4001
(800) 223-1138

American Diabetes Association (ADA)—For information on upcoming ADA events, publications, and local affiliates
1660 Duke St.
Alexandria, VA 22314
(800) DIABETES

National Diabetes Information Clearinghouse—For reading materials and updated information
1 Information Way
Bethesda, MD 20892–3560
(301) 654-3327

Circle of Life Camp, Inc.
Woodridge Dr.
Loudonville, NY 12211
(518) 459-3622

Diabetes Workshop, Inc.
2280 Western Ave.
Albany, NY 12084
(518) 862-1684

PERIODICALS

Countdown—A quarterly magazine, free with membership to a local JDF Chapter; $25 per year for membership and magazine
Juvenile Diabetes Foundation
    International
Editorial/World Headquaters
120 Wall St.
New York, NY 10005–4001
(800) 223-1138

Diabetes Forecast—A monthly magazine included with an ADA membership; $24 per year for membership and magazine
American Diabetes Association
1660 Duke St.
Alexandria, VA 22314
(800) 806-7801

Diabetes Interview—A monthly newspaper available by subscription; prices in US: 1 year $17.95; 2 years $29.95; 3 years $39.95; 5 years $49.95
Kings Publishing
3715 Balboa St.
San Francisco, CA 94121
(415) 387-4002

Diabetes Self-Management—A bimonthy magazine available by subscription; $18/1 year
Rapaport Publishing, Inc.
150 West 22nd St.
New York, NY 10011
(800) 234-0923

BOOKS

Understanding Insulin-Dependent Diabetes (The Pink Panther Book)— Twenty-five chapters cover all aspects of diabetes concerns. Easily understandable by the young adolescent and family.
Children's Diabetes Foundation at
    Denver
777 Grant St., Suite 302
Denver, CO 80203

FROM CHRONIMED PUBLISHING

Available at bookstores, or by calling (800) 848-2793:

In Control: A Guide for Teens with Diabetes by Jean Betschart, MN, RN, CDE, and Susan Thom, RD, LD, CDE. A highly readable guide that gives 12- to 18-year olds the facts they need to make the right choices about their health. A Juvenile Diabetes Foundation Library book.

It's Time to Learn About Diabetes: An Activity Book on Diabetes for Children by Jean Betschart, MN, RD, CDE. This workbook not only teaches elementary school-age children about what's happening to their bodies, but also helps them take care of themselves. A Juvenile Diabetes Foundation Library book.

Everyone likes to Eat by Hugo J. Hollerorth, EdD, and Debra Kaplan, RD, MS, with Anna Maria Bertorelli, MBA, RD, CDE. Written in conjunction with the Joslin Diabetes Center, this book shows how elementary school-age children can eat most of the foods they enjoy and still control diabetes.

Diabetes 101: A Pure and Simple Guide for People Who Use Insulin by Betty Page Brackenridge, MS, RD, CDE, and Richard O. Dolinar, MD. Written without complicated medical and technical jargon, this guide uses real-life examples in a story format to answer the questions every person with diabetes has.

Diabetes: A Guide to Living Well by Ernest Lowe and Gary Arsham, MD, PhD. A comprehensive book that helps readers design a program of individualized self-care that fits their lifestyle. Offers strategies for dealing with stress, emotional reactions, and difficult-to-change habits.

A Magic Ride in Foozbah-Land: An Inside Look at Diabetes by Jean Betschart, MN, RN, CDE. A fully illustrated adventure story that gives 3- to 7-year olds (and their parents) a better understanding of diabetes and how to manage it.

Juvenile Diabetes Foundation Chapters

For general information or assistance
in contacting the nearest JDF chapter,
call or write to:

Juvenile Diabetes Foundation
    International (JDF)
120 Wall St., 19th Floor
New York, NY 10005-4001
(800) 223-1138

ALABAMA
Birmingham Chapter
1442 Montgomery Highway, Suite 206
Birmingham, AL 35216
(205) 823-1907

ARKANSAS
First Arkansas Chapter
101 Fox Creek
Hot Springs, AR 71901
(501) 321-9182

ARIZONA
Arizona Chapter
1 East Camelback, Suite 605
Phoenix, AZ 85012
(602) 264-0370

CALIFORNIA
Inland Empire Chapter
1520 North Waterman Ave.
San Bernadino, CA 92404
(909) 888-3298

Los Angeles Chapter
1030 South Arroyo Parkway,
    Suite 204
Pasadena, CA 91105
(818) 403-1480

Orange County Chapter
1451 Quail St., Suite 108
Newport Beach, CA 92660
(714) 533-0363

Riverside County Chapter
5885 Brockton Ave.
Riverside, CA 92506
(909) 369-1392

Sacramento Valley Chapter
1121 Gold Country Blvd., Suite 106A
Gold River, CA 95670
(916) 635-2873

San Diego Chapter
8304 Clairemont Mesa Blvd.,
    Suite 101
San Diego, CA 92111
(619) 279-9160

Greater Bay Area Chapter
3641A Sacramento St.
San Francisco, CA 94118
(415) 441-7720

Monterey Bay Area Branch
225 Crossroads Blvd. Suite 326
Carmel, CA 93923
(408) 626-6254

COLORADO
Rocky Mountain Chapter
225 East 16th Ave., Suite 710
Denver, CO 80203
(303) 863-8940

Colorado Springs Branch
(719) 684-2230

Greeley Branch
(303) 353-3602

CONNECTICUT
Greater Hartford Chapter
18 North Main St., 3rd Floor
West Hartford, CT 06107
(860) 561-1153

Greater New Haven Chapter
364 Whitney Ave.
New Haven, CT 06511
(203) 776-3200

Fairfield Chapter
16 Forest St.
New Canaan, CT 06840
(203) 972-1729

DELAWARE
First State Chapter
3202 Kirkwood Highway, Suite 206
Wilmington, DE 19808
(302) 633-3350

DISTRICT OF COLUMBIA
Capitol Chapter
1400 "I" St. Northwest, Suite 500
Washington, DC 20005
(202) 371-0044

FLORIDA
South Florida Chapter
1415 East Sunrise Blvd., Suite 504
Fort Lauderdale, FL 33304
(954) 768-9008

Sarasota/Manatee Chapter
1765 Oak Lakes Drive
Sarasota, FL 34232
(941) 378-0801

Central Florida Chapter
266 Wilshire Blvd., Suite 151
Casselberry, FL 32707
(407) 331-2873

North Florida Chapter
830 Third St., Suite 108
Jacksonville Beach, FL 32250
(904) 249-3300

Palm Beach Chapter
204 Brazilian Ave., Suite 220
Palm Beach, FL 33480
(561) 655-0825

Greater Palm Beach County Chapter
3910 RCA Blvd., Suite 31011
Palm Beach Garden, FL 33410
(561) 625-6675

Tampa Bay Chapter
300 Third Ave. North, Suite 210
St. Petersburg, FL 33701
(813) 821-3588

GEORGIA
Georgia Chapter
235 Peachtree St., North East, #675
Atlanta, GA 30303
(404) 420-5990

HAWAII
Hawaii Chapter
733 Bishop St., Suite 2090
Honolulu, HI 96813
(808) 531-5698

ILLINOIS
Greater Chicago Chapter
500 North Dearborn, Suite 305
Chicago, IL 60610-4901
(773) 670-0313

INDIANA
Greater Indianapolis Chapter
6214 Morenci Trail, Suite 290
Indianapolis, IN 46268
(317) 329-9190

Northern Indiana Branch
PO Box 2195
Middlebury, IN 46540
(219) 875-1608

IOWA
Central Iowa Chapter
PO Box 4691
Des Moines, IA 50306-4691
(515) 967-6623

Siouxland Guild
3845 Jones St.
Sioux City, IA 51104
(712) 277-2700

KANSAS
Kansas City Chapter
6901 West 63rd, Suite 406
Shawnee Mission, KS 66202
(913) 831-7997

KENTUCKY
Louisville Chapter
1939 Goldsmith Lane, Suite 152
Louisville, KY 40218
(502) 485-9397

LOUISIANA
Louisiana Chapter
433 Metairie Rd., Suite 204
Metairie, LA 70005
(504) 828-2873

MAINE
Portland Chapter
PO Box 426
Westbrook, ME 04098
(207) 854-1810

MARYLAND
Maryland Chapter
5 E. Gwyns Mills Ct.
Owings Mills, MD 21117
(410) 356-4555

MASSACHUSETTS
Worcester County Chapter
PO Box 445
Greendale Station, MA 01606
(508) 829-3549

Bay State Chapter
20 Walnut St., Suite 201
Wellesley, MA 02181
(617) 431-0700

Greater Springfield Chapter
11 Acorn Lane
Ludlow, MA 01056
(413) 589-0687

MICHIGAN
Metropolitan Detroit Chapter
29350 Southfield Rd., Suite 42
Southfield, MI 48076
(810) 569-6171

Ann Arbor Branch
(313) 662-4708

Dearborn/ Downriver Branch
(313) 582-7520

West Michigan Chapter
4362 Cascade Rd. Southeast,
    Suite 116
Grand Rapids, MI 49546
(616) 957-1838

MINNESOTA
Hiawathaland Chapter
PO Box 6953
Rochester, MN 55903
(507) 288-7847

Minneapolis/St. Paul Chapter
2626 East 82nd St., Suite 230
Bloomington, MN 55425
(612) 851-0770

MISSISSIPPI
Southern Mississippi Chapter
RTE 5, Box 511
Brookhaven, MS 39601
(601) 366-4400

MISSOURI
St. Louis Chapter
225 South Meramec Ave., Suite 400
Clayton, MO 63105
(314) 726-67776

NEBRASKA
Lincoln Chapter
965 NBC Center
Lincoln, NE 68509
(402) 435-7663

Omaha Council Bluffs Chapter
7101 Newport Ave., Suite 209-F
Omaha, NE 68152-2153
(402) 572-3435

NEVADA
Nevada Chapter
4220 South Maryland Parkway,
    Suite 112
Las Vegas, NV 89119
(702) 732-4795

NEW HAMPSHIRE
New Hampshire Center
15 Tanguay Ave., Suite 114
Nashua, NH 03063
(603) 595-2595

NEW JERSEY
Cape Atlantic Chapter
c/o Argus Real Estate
6511 Ventnor Ave.
Atlantic City, NJ 08406
(609) 823-0689

Central Jersey Chapter
3430 Sunset Ave., Suite 21A
Ocean Township, NJ 07712
(908) 918-8455

North Jersey Chapter
513 W Mt. Pleasant Ave., Suite 225
Livingston, NJ 07039
(201) 992-0375

Rockland/Bergen/Passaic Chapter
560 Sylvan Ave.
Engelwood Cliffs, NJ 07632
(201) 568-4838

South Jersey Chapter
496 Kings Highway North
Cherry Hill, NJ 08034
(609) 779-9202

Mid-Jersey Chapter
2865 US Highway 1, Route 1,
   Finnegans Lane
North Brunswick, NJ 08902
(908) 422-9590

NEW YORK
Western New York Chapter
331 Alberta Dr., Suite 106
Amherst, NY 14226
(716) 833-2873

Rochester Branch
277 Alexander St., Suite 810
Rochester, NY 14607
(716) 546-1390

Dutchess County Branch
Edison Motor Inn, Route 55
Poughkeepsie, NY 12603
(914) 454-9458

Long Island/South Shore Chapter
PO Box 358
Cedarhurst, NY 11516
(516) 569-2200

Mid-Hudson Chapter
PO Box 157
Slate Hill, NY 10973-0157
(914) 355-1625

Long Island/Nassau Suffolk Chapter
364 Willis Ave.
Mineola, NY 11501-1500
(516) 739-2873

New York Chapter
381 Park Ave. South, Suite 507
New York, NY 10016
(212) 689-2860

Brooklyn Branch
(212) 689-2860

Staten Island Branch
(718) 727-5326

Queens Branch
(718) 478-1594

Westchester County Chapter
237 Mamaroneck Ave.
White Plains, NY 10605
(914) 696-7700

Capital-Saratoga Chapter
Greenwood Dr.
East Greenbush, NY 12061
(518) 477-2873

Syracuse Chapter
Box 71, Solvay Station
Syracuse, NY 13209
(315) 474-7011

Ulster County Chapter
PO Box 24
Lake Katrine, NY 12449
(914) 336-5426

NORTH CAROLINA
Asheville Guild
5 Arboretum Rd.
Asheville, NC 28803
(704) 274-3136

Piedmont Triad Chapter
632 Holly Ave.
Winston-Salem, NC 27101
(910) 724-2873

Charlotte Chapter
1012 South Kings Dr., Suite 701
Charlotte, NC 28283
(704) 377-2873

Triangle Chapter
183 Wind Chime Ct., Suite 201
Raleigh, NC 27615
(919) 870-5171

OHIO
Greater Cincinnati Chapter
10910 Reed Hartman Highway,
   Suite 202
Cincinnati, OH 45242-3828
(513) 793-3223

Cleveland Chapter
4500 Rockside Rd., Suite 420
Cleveland, OH 44131
(216) 524-6000

Greater Dayton Chapter
1281 H Lyons Rd.
Dayton, OH 45458
(513) 439-2873

Mid Ohio Chapter
1824 East Broad St.
Columbus, OH 43203
(614) 258-3398

East Central Ohio Chapter
4150 Belden Village St. NW,
   Suite 11-15
Canton, OH 44718
(330) 492-2873

Northwest Ohio Chapter
PO Box 367
Perrysburg, OH 43552
(419) 843-7787

OKLAHOMA
Central Oklahoma Chapter
3030 North West Expressway,
   Suite 1350
Oklahoma City, OK 73112
(405) 948-0004

Green County Guild
7101 South Yale, Suite 298
Tulsa, OK 74136
(405) 948-0004

OREGON
Greater Portland Chapter
8415 SW Seneca St., Suite 100
Tualatin, OR 97062
(503) 691-1995

PENNSYLVANIA
Berks County Chapter
Box 41, 2481 Lancaster Pike
Reading, PA 19607
(610) 775-4163

Central Pennsylvania Chapter
1104 Fernwood Ave., Suite 500
Camp Hill, PA 17011
(717) 730-0443

Lawrence County Chapter
RD 3 Box 16C
Volant, PA 16156
(412) 533-3545

Norristown Chapter
5108 Brandywine Dr.
Eagleville, PA 19403
(610) 630-1490

Philadelphia Chapter
225 City Line Ave., Suite 208
Bala Cynwyd, PA 19004
(610) 664-9255

Western Pennsylvania Chapter
300 Sixth Ave., Suite 260M
Pittsburgh, PA 15222
(412) 471-1414

Northwestern Pennsylvania Chapter
1673 West 8th St.
Erie, PA 16505
(814) 452-0635

SOUTH CAROLINA
Low Country Chapter
667 Ferry St.
Mt. Pleasant, SC 29464
(803) 766-0385

Palmetto Chapter
3608 Landmark Dr., Suite C
Columbia, SC 29204
(803) 782-1477

SOUTH DAKOTA
Sioux Falls Chapter
PO Box 88540
Sioux Falls, SD 57109-1003
(605) 338-2295

Watertown Chapter
107 Summerwood Dr.
Watertown, SD 57201
(605) 886-3777

TENNESSEE
East Tennessee Chapter
PO Box 91
Madisonville, TN 37354
(423) 442-3861

Greater Knoxville Chapter
433 Sevier Ave.
 #416 Rivermont Building
Knoxville, TN 37920
(423) 577-7530

Central Tennessee Chapter
2200 Hillsboro, Suite 110
Nashville, TN 37212
(615) 383-6781

TEXAS
Dallas Chapter
9400 N Central Expressway,
 Suite 903
Dallas, TX 75231
(214) 373-9808

Tarrant County Branch
601 Bailey Ave.
Fort Worth, TX 76107
(817) 332-2601

Houston Gulf Coast Chapter
5075 Westheimer, Suite 682
Houston, TX 77056
(713) 965-9742

West Texas Chapter
PO Box 7308
Midland, TX 79708
(915) 684-0902

South Central Texas Chapter
4115 Medical Dr., Suite 202
San Antonio, TX 78229-5635
(210) 692-9264

UTAH
Utah Chapter
320 West 200 South, Suite 170-B
Salt Lake City, UT 84101
(801) 530-0660

VIRGINIA
Roanoke Valley Chapter
3201 Brandon Ave., Southwest,
 Suite 5
Roanoke, VA 24018
(540) 345-8193

Southside VA Chapter
725 Tuscarora Dr.
Danville, VA 24540
(804) 793-4133

WASHINGTON
Seattle Chapter
Tillicum Marina, 1333 N. Northlake
 Way, Suite G
Seattle, WA 98103
(206) 545-1510

Seattle Guild
1001 4th Ave., Suite 3808
Seattle, WA 98154
(206) 343-0873

Spokane County Area Chapter
W. 422 Riverside Ave., Suite 1411
Spokane, WA 99201
(509) 459-6307

WEST VIRGINIA
Huntington Chapter
PO Box 2903
Huntington, WV 25728-2903
(304) 525-6721

WISCONSIN
Fox Valley Chapter
105 High St., Room 110
Neenah, WI 54956
(414) 725-1004

Greater Madison Chapter
PO Box 46039
Madison, WI 53744
(608) 836-4408

Milwaukee Chapter
2323 North Mayfair Rd., Suite 104
Wauwatosa, WI 53226
(414) 453-4673

CANADA
JDF Canada
98 Granton Dr.
Richmond Hill
Ontario L4B 2N5 Canada
(905) 889-4171

acceptance of diabetes
  independence, 94
  parental, 4–5
  parents vs. children, 6
adjustment to diabetes
  acceptance of, 6
  children's pain vs. parents' pain,
    8–9
  helplessness, 8
  loss of control, 8
  sibling's support and involvement,
    10–11
adolescents
  accepting diabetes, 93–94
  decision-making and indepen-
    dence, 92–93
  education and, 33
  physical changes for, and effect
    on diabetes, 79
American Diabetes Association's
  National Youth Congress, experience of, 55–56
American Diabetes Association, xii
  for social interaction, 59
anger
  of children, 6
  diagnosis and, 4–5
blood sugar. See also glucose level
  carbohydrate content and, 26
  importance of control of, 25

candy, 26
carbohydrate counting, 77
  sneaking food and, 34–35
carbohydrates, content and blood
  sugar, 26
Circle of Life Camp, Inc., xii–xiii, 4
  See also diabetes camps
  atmosphere of, 61
  benefits of, 60–61
  formation of, 59
  independence and, 86
  philosophy of, 60
  soccer game skit, 37
Control Diabetes Services, Inc., xii

dating, education and, 31–32
decision-making, independence and,
  92–93
denial, 15
  of children, 6
diabetes
  adjustment to, 6
  chronic condition vs. disease, xv
  complications associated with, xv
  misconceptions of, 21–22, 47, 75
  organizations and resources for,
    99–100
  using as excuse, 48
diabetes camps. See also Circle of
  Life Camp, Inc.
  benefits of, 62
  convincing child to attend, 63

importance of, 56
independence and, 86
misconceptions of, 56
parent's letting go, 63–64
Diabetes Complications and Control
  Trials, 25
diabetes management habits
  discipline and, 50
  increasing child's responsibility
    over, 91–92
  individual variability and, 81–82
  rebellion and, 50–51
Diabetes Workshop, Inc., xii
  services of, 38–39
diabetic, 47
  damage of labeling as, 36–37
  identity and, 36–38
  stereotype of, 37
diagnosis of diabetes
  of author, 5–6, 56–57
  parents' feelings and, 4–5
discipline
  building responsibility and inde-
    pendence with, 48–50
  diabetes management habits, 50
  normalcy and, 47–50
  using diabetes as excuse, 48
doctor. See physician

eating disorders, 78–79
education
  age-appropriate, 24, 33, 39
  of child's schoolmates, 27–31
  of child, 24–27
  continuous, 33, 40
  Diabetes Workshop, Inc., 38–39
  of family, 22–24
  importance of, 12, 22, 27, 40
  independence and, 88
  misconception about diabetes and,
    47

positive changes from, 57
  for siblings, 12
Emerson, Ralph Waldo, 69
emotions
  anger, 6
  denial, 6, 15
  guilt, 12–16
  helplessness, 8
  parents' sensitivity to children's, 7

family
  diabetes effect on, 10–12
  education of, 22–24
  as safety net, 14–15
food issues
  carbohydrate counting, 77
  deprivation, 76–77
  eating disorders, 78–79
  eating sweets, 26
  parental nagging, 77–78
  sneaking food, 26, 34–35, 90
friends, education of, 27–31

glucose level
  carbohydrate content and, 26
  importance of control of, 25
  value judgments and, 26–27
glucose level, high
  child's guilt and, 81
  difficulty controlling, 69–72
  long-term impact of, 25
  physical effect and, 71–72
  stress and, 80–81
  troubleshooting, 80–81
glucose level, low, 73–74
  frustration over, 73–74
  nighttime, 73
Goethe, Johann W., 43
guilt
  dealing with, 12–16
  high glucose level and, 81

health professionals, frustrating
medical
   advise from, 72–73
Huxley, Aldous, 69
hyperglycemia
   child's guilt and, 81
   difficulty controlling, 69–72
   long-term impact of, 25
   physical effect and, 71–72
   stress and, 80–81
   troubleshooting, 80–81
hypoglycemia
   educating school faculty and,
      29–30
   frustration over, 73–74
   nighttime, 73
   symptoms of, 77–78
identity, as "diabetic", 36–38
independence
   acceptance of diabetes and, 94
   age-appropriate education, 33
   building trust, 90–95
   child's education of school faculty,
      31
   continuous education, 33
   decision-making, 92–93
   definition of, 85
   diabetes camp, 86
   discipline and, 49
   education and, 88
   forgetting about diabetes, 86
   increasing responsibility and,
      91–92
   letting go, 87–90
   overdependence and encouraging,
      93
   rewards and, 89
insulin pump, 73, 75–76

Juvenile Diabetes Foundation
   chapters, 101–106
   for social interaction, 59

Kaleidoscope, xii, 23

letting go, 73–74, 87–90
   diabetes camp and, 63–64

media, diabetes portrayal in, 21
Miller, Henry, 3
misconceptions of diabetes, 21–23,
   47, 75

nighttime hypoglycemia, 73
normalcy
   day-by-day approach, 44
   definition of, 43
   discipline, 47–50
   education on misconceptions of
      diabetes, 47
   full participation in activities,
      46–47
   incorporating diabetes into child's
      lifestyle, 44
   overcoming obstacles, 51–52
   parent's preoccupation with
      diabetes, 44–46
   using diabetes as excuse, 48
parents
   education of, 23–24
   letting go, 63–64, 73–74, 87–90
   nagging and food issues, 77–78
   negative attitude of, and effect on
      children, 16
Peer Counseling and Classroom and
   Faculty Education Program, 57
physician
   child's comfort with, 38
   choosing, 38
   communication with child, 39
Pink Panther Book, 28

puberty. See also adolescents
  physical changes during, and
    effect on diabetes, 79
rebellion, 33, 44, 47
  solutions for, 50–51
responsibility
  carbohydrate counting, 34
  discipline and, 49–50
  identity as diabetic and, 36–38
  increasing, and independence,
    91–92
  self-pity and, 35–36
  setting goals and, 34
  sneaking food, 34–35
rewards, 80
  at camp, 89
  importance of, 80
  independence and, 89
  for tireless efforts, 80
Roosevelt, Eleanor, 55, 85

school faculty
  child's responsibility and interac-
    tions with, 31
  education of, 27–31
  hypoglycemia, 29–30
  snack time and, 29
schoolmates, education of, 27–31
self-pity, child's feeling of, and
  responsibility building, 35–36
Seneca, 55
siblings
  education for, 12
  jealousy of, 11
  special attention for, 11
  support and involvement, 10–11
sneaking food, 90
  carbohydrate counting and, 34–35
stress, high glucose level and, 81
Sugar Free Gang, The, xii

support groups
  benefit of, 58
  importance of, 56
  misconceptions of, 56
  for parents, 59
  social interaction in, 59
sweets, eating, 26
Swindoll, Charles, 21